Contents

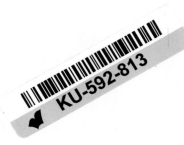

Models and Frameworks for Implementing Evidence-Based Practice

Linking Evidence to Action

Edited by

Jo Rycroft-Malone RN, MSc, BSc(Hons), PhD
Professor of Health Services & Implementation Research
Bangor University

and

Tracey Bucknall RN, ICU Cert, BN, Grad Dip Adv Nurs, PhD
Professor, School of Nursing Deakin University &
Head Cabrini-Deakin Centre for Nursing Research Cabrini
Health

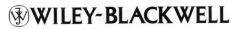
WILEY-BLACKWELL

A John Wiley & Sons, Ltd., Publication

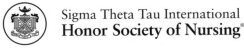
Sigma Theta Tau International
Honor Society of Nursing®

Library of Congress Cataloging-in-Publication Data

Models and frameworks for implementing evidence-based practice : linking evidence to action / edited by Jo Rycroft-Malone and Tracey Bucknall.
p. ; cm.
Includes bibliographical references and index.
ISBN 978-1-4051-7594-4 (pbk. : alk. paper)
1. Evidence-based nursing. I. Rycroft-Malone, Jo. II. Bucknall, Tracey.
[DNLM: 1. Evidence-Based Nursing—methods. 2. Models, Nursing.
WY 100.7 M689 2010]
RT84.5.M625 2010
610.73—dc22
2009040321

A catalogue record for this book is available from the British Library.

Set in 11/13 Sabon by MPS Limited, A Macmillan Company

Printed and bound in Malaysia by Vivar Printing Sdn Bhd

1   2010

Notes on Contributors

Tracey Bucknall

Tracey Bucknall RN, ICU Cert, BN, Grad Dip Adv Nurs, PhD is Professor in School of Nursing, Deakin University and Head, Cabrini-Deakin Centre for Nursing Research, Cabrini Health, and Associate Editor of *Worldviews on Evidence Based Nursing*. Tracey's primary research interests are clinical decision making and implementation of research into practice. Her research focuses on understanding how individuals make decisions routinely and in uncertainty, the environmental and social influences encountered in changing contexts, and interventions to improve the uptake of research in practice. More recently she has incorporated patient involvement in decision making as a means of influencing clinician uptake of research evidence.

Kara DeCorby

Kara DeCorby MSc is a research coordinator in the Faculty of Health Sciences at McMaster University. Kara has worked on several research projects related to knowledge translation and uptake; specifically promoting evidence-informed practice in public health decision making. She led the process of locating, relevance testing, key wording, and critical appraisal of reviews, in addition to summarizing review evidence and methodology in the development of http://www.health-evidence.ca, a registry of systematic review-level evidence on the effectiveness of public health interventions. Kara holds a clinical faculty appointment and cotutors a School of Nursing course on research methods and critical appraisal for primary studies and systematic literature reviews.

Maureen Dobbins

Maureen Dobbins RN, PhD is an Associate Professor and Career Scientist, Ontario Ministry of Health and Long-Term Care and is also associated with School of Nursing, McMaster University, Ontario, Canada. Her research is focused on understanding knowledge translation and exchange among public health decision makers in Canada. Studies have included: identification of barriers and facilitators to knowledge translation and exchange; understanding the information needs of public health decision makers; evaluating the use of systematic reviews in provincial policies; exploring where research evidence fits into the decision-making process; evaluating the impact of knowledge translation and exchange strategies; and exploring the role of knowledge brokers in facilitating evidence informed public health decision making.

Ellen Fineout-Overholt

Ellen Fineout-Overholt PhD, RN, FNAP, FAAN is Clinical Professor and Director at Arizona State University Center for the Advancement of Evidence-based Practice, AZ, USA. Dr. Fineout-Overholt has 20 years of combined experience as a critical care nurse, advanced practice nurse, researcher, and educator. Her program of research is developing and testing models of evidence-based practice in a variety of settings. Dr. Fineout-Overholt is coeditor of the recurring section, *Teaching EBP*, in Wiley-Blackwell and Sigma Theta Tau International's journal *Worldviews on Evidence-based Nursing*. In addition, she is coeditor of the number one selling book on EBP published by Lippincott Williams & Wilkins entitled, *Evidence-Based Practice in Nursing & Healthcare: A Guide to Best Practice*. In recognition of her contributions to professional nursing practice, Dr. Fineout-Overholt was inducted as a fellow in the National Academies of Practice in 2006 and the American Academy of Nursing in 2008.

Ian D Graham

Ian D Graham PhD is Vice-President of Knowledge Translation at the Canadian Institutes of Health Research and an Associate Professor in the School of Nursing at the University of Ottawa, Canada. Ian Graham has a PhD in medical sociology from McGill University. His research focuses on knowledge translation science and conducting applied research on the determinants of research use, strategies to increase implementation of research findings and evidence-based practice, and KT theories and models.

Jo Logan

Jo Logan is BScN and a PhD in Education. Jo Logan's interest in evidence-based practice began while teaching in hospital nursing staff development and extended to her position as Director of Nursing Research. Her efforts toward research utilization include the codevelopment and application of the Ottawa model of research use. The model was refined when Jo joined the University of Ottawa, School of Nursing. Her research interests focused on the foundations of evidence-based nursing. Currently, she holds a position as Adjunct Nursing Professor at the University of Ottawa.

Bernadette Mazurek Melnyk

Bernadette Mazurek Melnyk PhD, RN, CPNP/NPP, FNAP, FAAN is Dean and Distinguished Foundation Professor in Nursing at Arizona State University College of Nursing and Health Innovation and Associate Editor of *Worldviews on Evidence-Based Nursing*. Dr. Melnyk is a nationally/internationally recognized researcher, educator, clinician, speaker, and expert in evidence-based practice as well as in child and adolescent mental health. Her record of scholarship includes over 120 publications, including two books entitled *Evidence-Based Practice in Nursing & Healthcare: A Guide to Best Practice* and the *KySS Guide to Child and Adolescent Mental Health Screening, and Early Intervention and Health Promotion*. Dr. Melnyk has received numerous national/international awards and is a current member of the United States Preventive Services Task Force.

Alan Pearson

Alan Pearson RN, PhD, FRCNA, FAAG, FRCN is Executive Director at The Joanna Briggs Institute and Professor of Evidence Based Healthcare, The University of Adelaide, Australia. Professor Alan Pearson has extensive experience in nursing practice, nursing research, and academic nursing. He has practiced in the fields of orthopedics, maternal, child and community health and aged care in the United Kingdom, Papua New Guinea, and Australia. Professor Pearson has been an active researcher since 1981, known internationally for his pioneering work on the establishment and evaluation of nursing beds in Oxford, UK from 1981 to 1986 and for his ongoing work emphasizing the centrality of practice and evidence-based practice. He founded the Joanna Briggs Institute in 1996 and developed the *JBI Model of Evidence-Based Healthcare* with colleagues, in 2005.

Jo Rycroft-Malone

Jo Rycroft-Malone RN, MSc, BSc(Hons), PhD is Professor of Health Services and Implementation Research, Bangor University, UK and Editor of *Worldviews on Evidence-Based Nursing*. Jo's particular expertise and interests lie in knowledge translation research and evidence-based practice processes. She has successfully obtained national and international level competitive grants to study the processes and outcomes of evidence into practice interventions in a wide variety of topics. She is also a member of the PARIHS framework group. She sits on a number of national and international strategy development and funding groups including the National Institute for Health and Clinical Excellence (NICE) Implementation Strategy Group and the Canadian Institutes for Health Research Knowledge Exchange and Translation Committee. Jo is the inaugural editor of *Worldviews on Evidence-Based Nursing.*

Cheryl B Stetler

Cheryl B Stetler PhD, RN, FAAN. For over 25 years, Dr. Stetler worked in the acute care setting in a variety of positions, where she often was involved in implementing, conceptualizing, and evaluating research utilization/evidence-based practice and other change programs. Currently she is an international consultant on evidence-based practice and evaluation, providing consultation to, for example, the Veterans Administration QUERI Program; and is a Research Associate at the Boston University School of Public Health in Boston, MA, USA. Overall, her focus is the conceptualization and implementation of research utilization/evidence-based practice with a particular emphasis upon theory and organizational institutionalization of EBP into routine professional practice.

Marita Titler

Marita Titler PhD, RN, FAAN, is Professor, Associate Dean for Practice and Clinical Scholarship Development and the Rhetaugh Dumas Endowed Chair, University of Michigan School of Nursing, MI, USA. Marita's program of research focuses on translation science, interventions to improve outcomes of adults with chronic illnesses, and dissemination of evidence-based practice guidelines for the elderly. She has held multimillion dollar grants to study translation practice across a variety of topics including pain management and falls prevention. She is currently a member of the Institute of Medicine Forum on the Science of Health Care Quality Improvement and Implementation, the AHRQ HCTDS study section and the Appalachian Regional Healthcare, Board of Trustees, and is a fellow in the American Academy of Nursing. She has published widely and spoken nationally and internationally on evidence-based practice.

Paula Robeson

Paula Robeson BN, MScN, is Knowledge Broker (KB), health-evidence. ca (H-E) at McMaster University, Canada. As the KB, Paula plays an integral role in the delivery of services and resources to Canadian public health decision makers. In particular, she conducts tailored organizational, divisional, or team assessments of capacity for evidence-informed decision making with practical recommendations for action; provides customized knowledge brokering services to mentor individuals or teams in their efforts to incorporate the best available evidence in their practice, programs, and policy decisions; facilitates standard and tailored workshops and presentations addressing the "how to's" of evidence-informed practice; responds to practice-based questions and requests for evidence that are posted on the H-E website.

Jacqueline M Tetroe

Jacqueline M Tetroe MA, Knowledge Translation Portfolio, Canadian Institutes of Health Research, Ottawa, Canada. Jacqueline has a Masters Degree in developmental psychology and studied cognitive and educational psychology at the Ontario Institute for Studies in Education. She currently works as a senior advisor in knowledge translation at the Canadian Institutes of Health Research. Her research interests focus on the process of knowledge translation and on strategies to increase the uptake and implementation of evidence-based practice as well as to increase the understanding of the barriers and facilitators that impact on successful implementation. She is a strong advocate of the use of conceptual models to both guide and interpret research.

Foreword

Around the globe, huge expenditure supports a veritable industry of research to underpin evidence in health care. Studies on diagnostics, prognostics, and therapeutics provide ever finer-grained understandings about the nature of ill health, its assessment, potential causal pathways, likely trajectory and scope for amelioration. A more recent elaboration of this industry has been the many and varied attempts to collate, synthesis, and integrate the findings from diverse research into "evidence," with the hope that such evidence will be "implemented" by health-care practitioners for the betterment of patient care. Of course, both "evidence" and "implementation" are tricky customers that elude neat and consensual definitions (of which more later), but the central concern of this book is that we have an abundance of evidence alongside a relatively impoverished view of implementation. The stubborn and widespread failure of health-care practice to align with best evidence is a testimony to the rightness of this concern.

Dominating thinking on evidence-based practice – often implicitly – is a poorly expressed combination of cybernetics alongside notions of cognitive behavioral change. Too often, the emphasis has been on the proper and rigorous processes for the creation of evidence (systematic reviews, guidelines, clinical pathways, best-practice statements), and the promulgation of these through health systems, organizations and the professions (dissemination strategies of one form or another). Such dissemination may then be accompanied both by attempts to skill-up individual health-care practitioners in evidence use (seeking, appraising, applying, etc.), and by systems of audit and accountability for evidence uptake and impact (measuring and monitoring, and sometimes incentivizing, process measures of change). The problem to which this book addresses itself is that these latter activities (dissemination, implementation, impact assessment) are poorly or even erroneously conceptualized, underresourced, underresearched and, in short, somewhat neglected.

It is a real pleasure to see drawn together some of the better work on implementation that has unfolded over the past two decades and sometimes more. The theories, models, and frameworks presented here, often by some of their progenitors, provide a timely antidote to the narrowness of view that cybernetics and cognitive behavioral change are the sole (or even primary) engines of implementation. While earlier models presented may have their roots in individual-level change, more recent elaborations – or indeed, newer models – often take a broader view of multilevel change, seeing it as operating at individual, team, and organization levels. And while evidence is obviously an important component in each of the models, the social and contextual understandings of this evidence are brought to the fore in many, and evidence-use becomes conceptualized as a complex, socially situated process.

The plethora of theories, models, and frameworks available, and the careful laying out of the relative strengths, challenges, and scope for application, provides for the first time a comprehensive overview of not just ways of thinking about implementation, but also guidance on the practical application of these ways of thinking. Moreover, the editors have been careful to ensure good read-across between chapters (allowing easy comparison of convergence and divergence between models) and have taken the trouble to synthesize some of the key features of the models in a couple of useful concluding chapters. After all this careful laying out of the tools available, there is now no excuse among managers and practitioners for any lack of explicit underpinnings to any implementation effort.

If there is a criticism of the models presented in this book, it is that most take a "research into practice" view, where the task is conceived of as the application of preexisting knowledge in new contexts. Yet, as alluded to in the opening paragraph, "evidence" may not be so static a resource as that, and reducing research "implementation" to a simple matter of "doing the right thing" may undersell its contribution. Indeed, evidence may be created (or cocreated) as much in the process of implementation as it exists outside of that process. While these challenges are taken up in, for example, the knowledge to action framework, many of the models take a rather more unproblematic view of evidence and its use. Of course, such a criticism should be seen in context: much of the evidence base now available in health care is indeed of the instrumentalist kind. Although a critical understanding of how such evidence is received and constructed is important, the practical challenges may well come down to issues of application of that evidence in practice, challenges to which these models are well suited.

Kurt Lewin (1890–1947), recognized as one of the founders of social psychology, noted that "there is nothing so practical as a good theory" (1951: 169). This book provides a rich demonstration of that assertion. It will be invaluable not only to nurses and other health-care practitioners interested in more nuanced and better conceptualized understandings of implementation, but also to all those interested in the role of theories for understanding knowledge-informed change. It is to be hoped that it is used not only to inform new implementation strategies, but also to inform new investigative efforts on the success or otherwise of those strategies. Theories, models, and frameworks retain their vitality only in as much as they are invigorated through the application of fresh data.

Huw Davies
Professor of Health Care Policy & Management
University of St Andrews

and

Director, Knowledge Mobilisation & Capacity Building for
The UK's National Institute for Health Research (NIHR) Service
Delivery and Organisation (SDO) National Research Programme

Reference

Lewin, K. (1951). *Field theory in social science: Selected theoretical papers.* D. Cartwright (ed.). New York: Harper & Row.

Preface

This book and book series emerged from many discussions between us about the lack of resources that specifically consider the *implementation* of evidence into practice. Governments in developed countries across the world have made considerable investments in an infrastructure to support evidence generation (e.g., clinical guideline development, production of systematic reviews) but much less investment in evidence implementation. Arguably the political focus on evidence generation has been at the expense of implementation of that evidence. For example, when a national clinical guideline has been developed – there is often little or no consideration of the implementation implications of the practice recommendations contained within it. Furthermore, there has been a focus on developing the skills and knowledge of individual practitioner's to appraise research and make rational decisions using this knowledge in practice. We believe that while critical appraisal is an important skill, it is not sufficient for using evidence in day-to-day practice. Using evidence in practice is a complex process (not a one-off event), which requires more than a focus on individual factors. The implementation of evidence-based practice depends on an ability to achieve significant and planned change involving individuals, teams, and organizations.

When we did some research on what resources are available to guide and support implementation, we were surprised by how few there are. While there are many books under the umbrella of "evidence-based practice," these tend to take readers through the critical appraisal and research process, with extremely limited coverage of implementation issues. This book, one in a series of three to be published in parallel, aims to redress this imbalance.

The objective of this book is to consider the use of theory, models, and frameworks in the implementation of evidence-based practice, provide a collection of models and frameworks written by their developers, and offer a review and synthesis of these. Our intention is to provide a useful resource to help readers make decisions about the appropriateness of the various models' and frameworks' use in implementation efforts, and to inform theory use and development in the field more generally.

Jo Rycroft-Malone
Tracey Bucknall

Chapter 1

Evidence-based practice
Doing the right thing for patients

Tracey Bucknall and Jo Rycroft-Malone

Introduction

Profound changes in health care have occurred as a result of advances in technology and scientific knowledge. Although these developments have improved our ability to achieve better patient outcomes, the health system has struggled to incorporate new knowledge into practice. This partly occurs because of the huge volume of new knowledge available that the average clinician is unable to keep abreast of the research evidence being published on a daily basis. A commonly held belief is that knowledge of the correct treatment options by clinicians will lead more informed decision making and therefore the correct treatment for an individual. Yet the literature is full of examples of patients receiving treatments and interventions that are known to be less effective or even harmful to patients. Although clinicians genuinely wish to do the right thing for patients, Reilly (2004) suggests that good science is just one of several components to influence health professionals. Faced with political, economic, and sociocultural considerations, in addition to scientific knowledge and patients' preferences, decision making becomes a question of what care is appropriate for which person under what circumstances. Not surprisingly, to supplement to clinical expertise, critical appraisal has become an important prerequisite for all clinicians (nurses, physicians, and allied health) to evaluate and integrate the evidence into practice.

Although there is the potential to offer the best health care to date, many problems exist that prevent the health care system from delivering up to its potential. Globally, we have seen continuous escalation of health care costs, changes in professional and nonprofessional roles and accountability related to widespread workforce shortages, and limitations placed on the accessibility and availability of resources. A further development has been the increased access to information via multimedia, which has promoted greater involvement of consumers in their treatment and management. This combination has lead to a focus on improving the quality of health care universally and the evolution of evidence-based practice (EBP).

What is evidence-based practice?

Early descriptions simply defined EBP as the integration of best research evidence with clinical expertise and patient values to facilitate clinical decision making (Sackett *et al.*, 2000: 1). The nursing society, Sigma Theta Tau International 2005–2007 Research & Scholarship Advisory Committee (2008) further delineated evidence-based nursing as "an integration of the best evidence available, nursing expertise, and the values and preferences of the individuals, families, and communities who are served" (p.69). However, an early focus on using the best evidence to solve patient health problems oversimplified the complexity of clinical judgment and failed to acknowledge the contextual influences such as the patient's status or the organizational resources available that change constantly and are different in every situation.

Haynes *et al.* (2002) expanded the definition and developed a prescriptive model for evidence-based clinical decisions. Their model focused on the individual and health care provider and incorporated the following: the patient's clinical state, the setting and circumstances; patient preferences and actions; research evidence; and clinical expertise. Di Censo *et al.* (2005) expanded the model further to contain four central components: the patient's clinical state, the setting and circumstances; patient preferences and actions; research evidence; and a new component *health care resources*, with all components overlaid by clinical expertise (Fig. 1.1). This conceptualization has since been incorporated into a new international position statement about EBP (STTI, 2008). This statement broadens out the concept of evidence further to include other sources of robust information such as audit data. It also includes key concepts of knowledge creation and distillation, diffusion and dissemination, and adoption, implementation, and institutionalization.

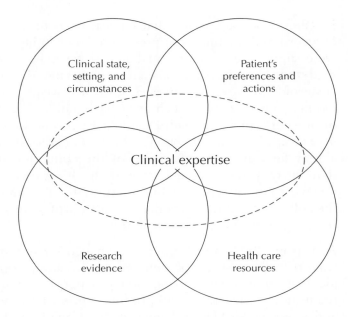

Figure 1.1 The interrelationship between evidence-based practice and clinical expertise (reprinted from Di Censo *et al.*, 2005, with permission from © 2005 Elsevier)

These changes to definitions and adaptations to models highlight the evolutionary process of EBP, from a description of clinical decision making to a guide that informs decisions. While there is an emphasis on a combination of multiple sources of information to inform clinicians' decision making in practice, it remains unknown how components are weighted and trade-offs made for specific decisions.

The evolution of evidence-based practice

A British epidemiologist, Archie Cochrane, was an early activist for EBP. In his seminal work, Cochrane (1972) challenged the use of limited public funding for health care that was not based on empirical research evidence. He called for systematic reviews of research so that clinical decisions were based on the strongest available evidence. Cochrane recommended that evidence be based on randomized controlled trials (RCTs) because they were more reliable than other forms of evidence. Research reviews should be systematically and rigorously prepared and updated regularly to include new evidence. These principles resonated with both the public and health care providers.

In 1987, Cochrane noted that clinical trials on the effectiveness of corticosteroid treatments in premature labor in high-risk pregnancies were supportive of treatment but had never been comprehensively analyzed. He referred to a systematic review that indicated corticosteroid therapy could reduce low-birth-weight premature infant mortality rates by 20% (Cochrane Collaboration, 2009). In recognition of his work and leadership, the first Cochrane Centre was opened 4 years after his death; the Cochrane Collaboration was founded a year later in 1993. The aim of the collaboration is to ensure that current research evidence in health care is systematically reviewed and disseminated internationally. Beginning in medicine, the collaboration now has many health professions represented on review groups including consumers.

As Kitson (2004) noted, the rise of evidence-based medicine (EBM) was in itself, a study of innovation diffusion, "offering a strong ideology, influential leaders, policy support and investment with requisite infrastructures and product" (p. 6). Early work by Sackett and team at McMaster University in Canada and Chalmers and team at Oxford in the UK propelled EBM forward, gaining international momentum. Since 1995, the Cochrane Library has published over 5000 systematic reviews, and has over 11,500 people working across 90 different countries (Cochrane Collaboration, 2009).

The application of EBM core principles spread beyond medicine and resulted in a broader concept of EBP. In nursing, research utilization (RU) was the term most commonly used from the early 1970s until the 1990s when EBP came into vogue. Estabrooks (1998) defined RU as "the use of research findings in any and all aspects of one's work as a registered nurse" (p. 19). More recently, Di Censo *et al.* (2005) have argued that EBP is a more comprehensive term than RU. It includes identification of the specific problem, critical thinking to locate the sources, and determine the validity of evidence, weighting up different forms of evidence including the patients preferences, identification of the options for management, planning a strategy to implement the evidence, and evaluating the effectiveness of the plan afterwards (Di Censo *et al.*, 2005).

The emergence of EBP has been amazingly effective in a short time because of the simple message that clinicians find hard to disagree with, that is, where possible, practice should be based on up to date, valid, and reliable research evidence (Trinder and Reynolds, 2000). In Box 1.1, four consistent reasons for the strong emergence of

> **Box 1.1 The emergence of evidence-based practice (Trinder and Reynolds, 2000)**
>
> | | |
> |---|---|
> | Research–practice gap | Slow and limited use of research evidence. Dependence on training knowledge, clinical experience, expert opinion, bias and practice fads. |
> | Poor quality of much research | Methodologically weak, not based on RCTs, or is inapplicable in clinical settings. |
> | Information overload | Too much research, unable to distinguish between valid and reliable research and invalid and unreliable research. |
> | Practice not evidence-based | Clinicians continue to use harmful and ineffective interventions. Slow or limited uptake of proven effective interventions being available. |

EBP across the health disciplines are summarized by Trinder and Reynolds (2000).

It is worth noting, however, that while generally accepted as an idea "whose time has come," EBP is not without its critics. It is often challenged on the basis that it erodes professional status (as a way of "controlling" the professions), and as a reaction to the traditional hierarchy of evidence (see Rycroft-Malone, 2006 for a detailed discussion of these arguments).

Although significant investment has been provided to produce and synthesize the evidence, a considerably smaller investment has been made toward the implementation side of the process. As a consequence, we have variable levels of uptake across the health disciplines and minimal understanding of the effectiveness of interventions and strategies used to promote utilization of evidence.

What does implementation of evidence into practice mean?

In health care, there have been many terms used to imply the introduction of an innovation or change into practice such as quality improvement, practice development, adoption of innovation,

Box 1.2 What is meant by implementation?

Diffusion	Information is distributed unaided, occurs naturally (passively) through clinicians adoption of policies, procedures, and practices.
Dissemination	Information is communicated (actively) to clinicians to improve their knowledge or skills; a target audience is selected for the dissemination.
Implementation	Actively and systematically integrating information into place; identifying barriers to change, targeting effective communication strategies to address barriers, using administrative and educational techniques to increase effectiveness.
Adoption	Clinicians commit to and actually change their practice.

Source: Definitions adapted from Davis and Taylor-Vaisey (1997).

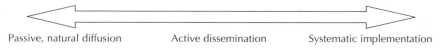

Passive, natural diffusion   Active dissemination   Systematic implementation

Figure 1.2 Nature of spread

dissemination, diffusion, or change management. The diversity in terminology has often evolved from the varying perspectives of those engaged in the activity such as clinicians, managers, policy makers, or researchers. Box 1.2 differentiates some of the definitions most frequently provided.

These definitions imply a continuum of implementation from the most passive form of natural diffusion after release of information toward more active dissemination where a target audience is selected and communicated the information to improve their skills and knowledge. Further along the continuum is the systematically planned, programed, and implemented strategy or intervention where barriers are identified and addressed and enablers are used to promote implementation for maximum engagement and sustainability (Fig. 1.2).

Implementation in health care has also been informed by many different research traditions. In a systematic review of the literature on diffusion, dissemination, and sustainability of innovations in health services, Greenhalgh *et al.* (2004) found 11 different research traditions that were relevant to understanding implementation in health care. These were: Diffusion of innovations; rural sociology; medical sociology; communication; marketing and economics; development studies; health promotion; EBM; organizational studies; narrative organizational studies; complexity and general systems theory. Box 1.3

Box 1.3 Examples of research traditions influencing diffusion, dissemination, and sustainable change

Research tradition	Findings
Diffusion of innovation	Innovation originates at a point and diffuses outward (Ryan, 1969).
Rural sociology	People copy and adopt new ideas from opinion leaders (Ryan and Gross, 1943).
Medical sociology	Innovations spread through social networks (Coleman *et al.*, 1966).
Communication	Persuading consumers while informing them (MacDonald, 2002). More effective if source and receiver share values and beliefs (MacGuire, 1978).
Marketing and economics	Persuading consumers to purchase a product or service. Mass media creates awareness; interpersonal channels promote adoption (MacGuire, 1978).
Development studies	Social inequities need to be addressed if widespread diffusion is to occur across different socioeconomic groups and lead to greater equity (Bourdenave, 1976).
Health promotion	Creating an awareness of the problem and offering a solution through social marketing. Messengers and change agents from target group increase success (MacDonald, 2002; Rogers, 1995).

(Continued)

Box 1.3 (Continued)

Research tradition	Findings
Evidence-based medicine	No causal link between the supply of information and its usage. Complexity of intervention and context influence implementation in real world (Greenhalgh *et al.*, 2004).
Organizational studies	Innovation as knowledge is characterized by uncertainty, immeasurability, and context dependence (Greenhalgh *et al.*, 2004).
Narrative organizational studies	Storytelling captures the complex interplay of actions and contexts; humanizing and sense-making, creating imaginative and memorable organizational folklore (Greenhalgh *et al.*, 2004; Gabriel, 2000).
Complexity and general systems	Complex systems are adaptive, self-organizing and responsive to different environments. Innovations spread via the local self-organizing interaction of actors and units (Plsek and Greenhalgh, 2001).

Source: Adapted from Greenhalgh *et al.* (2004).

outlines the research traditions and some key findings derived from the research.

The many different research traditions have used diverse research methods that at times produce contrasting results. For researchers, it offers significant flexibility in research design and depends on the research questions being asked and tested. For clinicians and managers, research theories offer guidance for developing interventions by exposing essential elements to be considered. These elements are often grouped at individual, organizational, and environmental levels, as they require different activities and strategies to address the element. The following section offers a limited review of the different attributes that are known to influence the success of implementation and need to be considered prior to implementing evidence into practice.

Attributes influencing successful implementation

Unlike the rapid spread associated with some forms of technology, which may simply require the intuitive use of a gadget and little persuasion to purchase it, many health care changes are complex interventions requiring significant skills and knowledge to make clinical decisions prior to integration into practice. Not surprisingly then, implementation of evidence into practice is mostly a protracted process, consisting of multiple steps, with varying degrees of complexity depending on the context. Numerous challenges arise out of the process that can be categorized into following five areas (Greenhalgh *et al.*, 2004): the evidence or information to be implemented, the individual clinicians who need to learn about the new evidence, the structure and function of health care organizations, the communication and facilitation of the evidence, and lastly, the circumstances of the patient who will be the receiver of the new evidence. These challenges need to be considered when tailoring interventions and strategies to the requirements of various stakeholders (Bucknall, 2006).

The evidence

There is much literature indicating that the characteristics of the evidence are an important consideration in planning implementation. Different types of evidence are known to spread at different rates. Characteristics of evidence include the type of evidence available to be implemented, the quality of the particular evidence, and the volume of evidence available to the decision maker such as a single RCT or a systematic review of multiple studies. These characteristics will all influence the rate, extent, and adherence of adoption by different individuals. In Rogers (1995) seminal works, he identified six major attributes of evidence that affect its uptake and sustained adoption. These included the *relative advantage* offered by the evidence to the patient or the clinician. First, clinicians must be able to clearly identify the benefits for patients or their own practice, either for improving patient outcomes, reducing harm, increasing access to resources, or decreasing costs. Second, the adopter's values and practices must be *compatible* with the evidence. Third, the more *complex* the evidence, the more difficult it will be for the clinician to use and to integrate into practice. Fourth, the degree to which the evidence can be tested on a limited basis, known as *trialability*, is important.

Trialing the evidence allows clinicians to practice and minimize any harmful or unexpected events associated with the implementation. Fifth, the adoption of evidence is also more likely when clinicians can *observe* others using the evidence; it provides some reassurance about the processes and minimization of harm for patients. Finally, to integrate the evidence into differing contexts, clinicians may need to *reinvent*, refine, or adapt the evidence to suit their own and their organizational needs (Rogers, 1995).

However, in their systematic review, Greenhalgh *et al.* (2004) argued that Roger's list of evidence attributes does not completely explain the adoption and adherence of complex health service innovations. New constructs have evolved from health service studies such as the importance of assessing the evidence in terms of relevance and usefulness for a specific task; the feasibility of implementing the change, the degree of implementation difficulty because numerous disciplines and specialties are involved; the ability to break the process into components to implement sections sequentially; and the prior knowledge and skills needed to use the evidence such as implementing new technology (Agarwal *et al.*, 1997; Greenhalgh *et al.*, 2004, Yetton *et al.*, 1999).

The individual clinician

Much early research paid close attention to characteristics of the individual in attempting to understand the reasons for the research–practice gap (Champion and Leach, 1989; Coyle and Sokop 1990; Estabrooks *et al.*, 2003; Rodgers, 2000). One of the challenges frequently identified is the prior knowledge and skills of the individual clinician. To assimilate the evidence into practice, clinicians need to be able to critically appraise the evidence to determine its validity and reliability. If they lack these basic educational skills then their ability to assess contradictory evidence and decide on the right course of action will be impaired (Bucknall, 2006; Bucknall *et al.*, 2008). Not only must clinicians weight the evidence, the volume may also require significant time to reflect and process the information. Again, this may depend on the ability of the individual as to the time taken to digest the information.

Personality traits such as motivation, learning styles, and the individual's capability will also determine adoption (Greenhalgh *et al.*, 2004). Wejnert (2002) suggested that depending on the organizational context at the time, the individual may assign greater meaning to the evidence and thus be more receptive to practice changes. The changing concerns and priorities, commonly associated with health care, may motivate different individuals at different stages throughout the process; each individual will have distinct personal makeup, knowledge and clinical experience, and as a consequence, unique concerns (Hall and Hord, 1987).

> To a greater or lesser extent (and differently in different contexts), individuals seek innovations out, experiment with them, evaluate them, find (or fail to find) meaning in them, develop feelings (positive or negative) about them, challenge them, worry about them, complain about them, work round them, talk to others about them, develop know-how about them, modify them to fit particular tasks, and attempt to improve or redesign them-often (and most successfully) through dialogue with other users. (Greenhalgh *et al.*, 2004: 163)

The health care organization

More recently, the failure of successful implementation in health care organizations has been attributed to the disregard shown toward organizational attributes or contextual factors. Organizational attributes are described as "those characteristics of health-care organizations, or units within those institutions, and of governance structures outside of those institutions that facilitate the dissemination and uptake of research findings" (Estabrooks, 1999: 61).

It is well recognized that organizations vary enormously within and between each other, hampering generalizability of research findings on implementation from one site or unit to the next. Indeed, the challenge for clinicians and managers is to overcome the structural determinants such as size, duration of establishment, degree of specialization, and decision-making structures known to influence knowledge transfer and uptake (Greenhalgh *et al.*, 2004). Greenhalgh *et al.'s* (2004) review showed that organizations were more likely to be successful at evidence integration if they have the capability to analyze, reframe, and combine the information with existing knowledge, that is, organizations with greater absorptive capacity. Organizations must also be receptive to change, taking risks, and experimenting with new evidence. The climate of the organization is shown to be fostered by strong leadership at managerial level and also within the clinical units (Bucknall, 2006). In addition, a culture of continuous learning is needed, appraising first and then using new knowledge and knowledge generated from monitoring changes, feeding back the information for refining the process within and across disciplines (Greenhalgh *et al.*, 2004).

Externally, informal interorganizational networks have been shown to be influential in successful practice change. It would appear though that a threshold proportion of organizations may be required to change before influencing others to do so. In contrast, an organizational network can be a negative effect that deters others from trying the change (Burns and Wholey, 1993; Valente, 1996) or stimulate a competitive environment (Castle, 2001). This has been useful in guideline implementation across quality improvement collaboratives when data is compared between organizations (Ovretveit *et al.*, 2002). Policy makers have been shown to have some influence although the success may be determined by the capacity to change (Fitzgerald *et al.*, 2002).

Communication and facilitation

In a classic study, Innvaer *et al.* (2002) reviewed 24 studies on research use by policy makers and found the primary facilitator and barrier of research use was personal contact (13/24) or lack thereof (11/24), respectively. Therefore, it comes as no surprise that communication with social contacts and networks have proven effective in transferring knowledge and increasing uptake of new evidence.

Four approaches have shown positive outcomes. The social network approach has been successful in different professional groups in health services. A social network is a group of people within a social system that provides friendship, advice, support, and communication (Valente, 1996). West *et al.* (1999) found that nurses had formal vertical networks whereas doctors had more informal horizontal networks. Vertical networks tend to cascade authoritative decisions more successfully, while horizontal networks wield greater influence during the reframing of evidence for local consumption (West *et al.*, 1999). In addition, there is greater success likely during implementation if the social network has similar educational, professional, and socioeconomic backgrounds (Rogers, 1995).

Change champions are another frequently used approach to endorse adoption of new evidence in organizations. Change champions are individuals who continually promote and support the use of new evidence within the group. Usually they are passionate experts, respected and informal leaders who have positive working relationships with other professionals (Greenhalgh *et al.*, 2004). Change champions can be placed at any level of the organization and provide differing roles.

The third approach for promoting practice change, influencing the actions and beliefs of their peers are opinion leaders (Locock *et al.*, 2001). Similar to change champions, opinion leaders operate at different levels of the organization. They can be internal, external, and peer opinion leaders. In general, opinion leaders are local, respected sources of influence trusted among their peer group to appraise new information and reframe it in the context of the local situation. They are accomplished in role modeling, influencing peers, and altering group norms (Rogers, 1995). Opinion leaders may also have a negative influence on the success of an intervention deterring their peers from using the evidence (Locock *et al.*, 2001).

A fourth approach for communicating evidence is through boundary spanners. Boundary spanners appraise and filter the evidence before disseminating it throughout the organization (Rogers, 1995). Their extensive social ties, both within and across organizations, link organizations experienced in the uptake of evidence to those yet to experience or in early stages of adoption.

The patient

Patient involvement in health care delivery can improve the success of implementation studies (Wensing *et al.*, 2005). From the early days of EBP, Sackett *et al.* (1996) argued that clinicians must take account of the patient's condition, baseline risk, values, and circumstances when making decisions about health care treatments. The inclusion of patient preferences into models of EBP demonstrates the growing support for patient involvement in health care decisions. The aim of involving patients in treatment decisions is to allow the patient to make health care decisions that accurately reflect their preferences and values (Bucknall, 2006). Benbassat *et al.* (1998) argued there is a lack of consistency by clinicians in assembling information on patient's values and preferences during treatment selection. Providers' beliefs of importance and what patients actually want may in fact be disparate. Similar to other individuals, patients are influenced by the type and stage of their illness, age, gender, culture, and socioeconomic status (Caress *et al.*, 1998; Pierce and Hicks, 2001). O'Connor *et al.* (1999) believe that health treatments always have advantages and disadvantages; therefore evidence alone cannot determine the best choice of treatment. Although the trade-offs for many clinical decisions are clear, there are occasions when there is a precarious balance between risks and benefits, and choices will differ across patients (O'Connor *et al.*, 1999).

Given we are all consumers of health care resources at some point in our lives, most of us would prefer the ability to choose the latest and most effective treatments and interventions to improve our situation. When patients have the capacity to understand and analyze information, they prefer a shared decision-making model (Degner *et al.*, 1997; Edwards and Elwyn, 2004).

The increased availability and accessibility to multimedia technology has ensured that patients and clients have increasing access to the same or similar information as clinicians. Searches of the Internet highlight the choices available for patients, potentially increasing their involvement in health management decisions and guiding the treatments administered by clinicians. Yet little is known about the role of the patient in promoting the rate of adoption among clinicians (Bucknall *et al.*, 2004; Wensing *et al.*, 2005). Patient-mediated interventions have been targeted at different stages: the decision to seek medical treatment and care; before and during contact with clinicians; and after care is delivered, for feedback on service (Wensing *et al.*, 2005). Greater responsiveness to patients may improve patient outcomes and the success of implementation.

Table 1.1 identifies the main elements and subelements that need to be considered during implementation of evidence into practice. It offers examples of questions for each subelement when planning an implementation strategy.

Why this book?

The application of knowledge into practice to improve patient care and outcomes is fundamental to health care. Yet our ability to translate knowledge into practice continues to be slow, fraught with challenges, and at times unsuccessful. The objective of this book is to provide a critical analysis of models and approaches for implementing

Table 1.1 Considerations for the successful implementation of evidence into practice

Element	Subelements	Questions for planning implementation
Evidence		
	Type of evidence	Is specific evidence available? Is it accessible? What is its quality?
		Does a relative advantage exist? Will patients benefit from receiving the EBP? Will anyone else benefit?
	Compatibility	How compatible is the evidence with practice?
	Complexity	How complex are the interventions? Are different levels of clinicians involved? Are different disciplines involved in the process? What do we need to change?
	Trialability	Can we trial different approaches to implement the same evidence? Can we adapt what we have or do we need a new approach?
	Observability	Can we see how others implement the evidence before we try it?
	Reinvention	Do we need to adapt the evidence to suit local conditions? How can we do this?
Clinician		
	Personality	What motivates the clinicians? What learning styles will be required to understand the evidence? What approach will best suit the clinician?
	Meaning	How important is the problem to the clinician?
	Independence	Can the clinician make the decision to implement or is permission needed?
Context		
	Structural determinants	What type of management structure is in place?
	Absorptive capacity	Who is responsible within the organization for analyzing and reframing the information suitable for local use? Is it a learning culture that fosters widespread interdisciplinary sharing of evidence?

(Continued)

Table 1.1 (*Continued*)

Element	Subelements	Questions for planning implementation
Communication and facilitation	Receptive to change	Is this evidence critical for the organization? Is there executive support for the change? Who is monitoring the change? What audit and feedback system is in place? What quality indicators are measured?
	Interorganizational networks	What interorganizational networks are in place to share information? Do these need to be built or fostered?
	Social networks	What approaches will foster evidence transfer and uptake? How might these be established or enhanced? Do different professions have different types? Is there sufficient interdisciplinary and specialty crossover?
	Homophily	What are the staff demographics of the organization?
	Change champions	Who are the likely change champions in the organization? Are they specialty change champions?
	Opinion leaders	What types of opinions leaders are contained within the organization? Are external opinions leaders present?
	Boundary spanners	Who is a likely boundary spanner? Does the organization have links with external boundary spanners? What professional groups need to be accessed?
Patients	Level of involvement	Does the patient wish to be involved? How could the patient be involved?
	Competence	Is the patient competent and able to be involved?
	Meaning	How important is the problem to the patient?
	Personality	What motivates the patient? What approach should be taken?

Source: Elements adapted from Rycroft-Malone *et al.* (2002), Greenhalgh *et al.* (2004), and Bucknall (2006)

EBP into a range of health care settings. In doing so, it will provide readers with a selection from which to choose the most appropriate model or approach to assist them in a successful implementation strategy for an assortment of evidence, individuals, and contexts.

While teaching EBP to students for more than a decade and in conducting implementation projects across health care settings, many barriers were encountered. In particular, the need to select a strategy suited to the type of evidence, the individuals involved and the local context were highlighted. In university courses, we gave students a range of models from which to select and develop a strategy for a change within their own practice setting. In making a selection, students offered critiques of alternative models and approaches, particularly in relation to their own skills, the resources available to them and the local context in which the change strategy needed to be applied. Not surprisingly, the selection and rationales for choosing models were widely varying and often difficult to make.

We have selected a range of models and frameworks that have been used internationally across settings from primary health to critical care. All these settings involve nurses and other health professionals working to deliver quality care to individuals with compromised or potentially compromised health and well-being. All the models have been subjected to external evaluation or testing and are potentially transferable across contexts. We have asked the authors of the chapters to provide background information on the type of model, the level at which it is best suited in application, the theoretical underpinnings, the settings the model has been used in and by which professional groups. Authors will summarize the testing and evaluation of the model as well as the practicalities and challenges in implementing the model in differing contexts. To conclude each chapter, authors will outline future research required in testing the model further.

Using the book

In identifying a gap in the resources to support planning and implementation of evidence into practice, we have structured the book to support international readers in their selection of an appropriate model for their local environment, to develop their understanding of its components, and more specifically to increase the uptake of evidence in practice.

Following the introduction, a chapter will take readers through existing knowledge translation theories and models in implementing EBP. The chapter will outline an approach to critically analyzing the selected models. Chapter 3 begins with one of the early models developed more than three decades ago in the USA by Stetler and Marram (1976). Chapters 3–10 will proceed through to the most recent models published in the literature, concluding with a Canadian framework, published 30 years after the original Stetler model.

In Chapter 11, we provide a narrative synthesis of all the models, integrating information to provide a useful summary and direction to people on the appropriateness of particular models for specific implementation issues and projects. The final chapter provides a summary and concludes with an outline of implications for implementing evidence into practice.

References

Agarwal, R., Tanniru, M., and Wilemon, D. (1997). Assimilating information technology innovations: Strategies and moderating influences. *Transactions on Engineering Management*, 44: 347–358.

Benbassat, J., Pilpel, D., and Tidhar, M. (1998). Patients' preferences for participation in clinical decision making: A review of published surveys. *Behavioral Medicine*, 24(2), 81–88.

Bourdenave, J.D. (1976). Communication of agricultural innovations in Latin America: The need for new models. *Communication Research*, 3: 135–154.

Bucknall, T.K. (2006). Knowledge transfer and utilization: Implications for home health care pain management. *Journal of Healthcare Quality*, 28(1): 12–19.

Bucknall, T.K., Rycroft-Malone, J., and Mazurek Melnek, B. (2004). Integrating patient involvement in treatment decisions (editorial). *Worldviews on Evidence-Based Nursing*, 1(3), 151–153.

Bucknall, T.K., Kent, B., and Manley, K. (2008). Evidence use and evidence generation in practice development. In K. Manley, B. McCormack, and V. Wilson (eds), *Practice Development in Nursing – International Perspectives*. London: Wiley Blackwell.

Burns, T. and Wholey, D.R. (1993). Adoption and abandonment of matrix management programs: Effects of organizational characteristics & inter-organizational networks. *Academy of Management Journal*, 36: 106–138.

Caress, A.-L., Luker, K.A., and Ackrill, P. (1998). Patient-sensitive treatment decision-making? Preferences and perceptions in a sample of renal patients. *NT Research*, 3(5): 364–372.

Castle, N.G. (2001). Innovations in nursing homes: Which facilities are the early adopters? *Gerontologist*, 41: 161–172.

Champion, V. L. and Leach, A. (1989). Variables related to research utilization in nursing: An empirical investigation. *Journal of Advanced Nursing*, 14(9), 705–710.

Cochrane, A. (1972). *Effectiveness and Efficiency: Random Reflections of Health Services*. London: Nuffield Provincial Hospitals Trust.

Cochrane Collaboration. (2009). Retrieved 23/07/09, from http://www.cochrane.org.

Coleman, J.S., Katz, E., and Menzel, H. (1966). *Medical Innovations: A Diffusion Study*. New York: Bobbs-Merrill.

Coyle, L.A. and Sokop, A.G. (1990). Innovation adoption behavior among nurses. *Nursing Research*, 39(3), 176–180.

Davis, D. and Taylor-Vaisey, A. (1997). Translating guidelines into practice: A systematic review of theoretic concepts, practical experience, and research evidence in the adoption of clinical practice. *Canadian Medical Association Journal*, 157: 408–416.

Degner, L.F., Kristjanson, L.J., Bowman, D., Sloan, J.A., Carriere, K.C., O'Neil, J., *et al.* (1997). Information needs and decision preferences in women with breast cancer. *JAMA,* 277(18): 1485–1492.

Di Censo, A., Guyatt, G., and Ciliska, D. (2005). *Evidence Based Nursing: A Guide to Clinical Practice* (Elsevier Health Sciences). London: Mosby, Inc.

Edwards, A. and Elwyn, G. (2004). The use of shared decision making skills and risk communication tools in common therapeutic decisions: A primary care trial. Retrieved June 8, 2004, from http://www.healthinpartnership.org/studies/edwards.html.

Estabrooks, C.A. (1998). Will evidence-based nursing practice make practice perfect? *Canadian Journal of Nursing Research*, 1(1), 15–36.

Estabrooks, C.A. (1999). Mapping the research utilization field in nursing. *Canadian Journal of Nursing Research*, 31(1), 53–72.

Estabrooks, C.A., Floyd, J.A., Scott-Findlay, S., O'Leary, K.A., and Gushta, M. (2003). Individual determinants of research utilization: A systematic review. *Journal of Advanced Nursing*, 43(5), 506–520.

Fitzgerald, L., Ferlie, E., Wood, M., and Hawkins, C. (2002). Interlocking interactions, the diffusion of innovations in health care. *Human Relations,* 55: 1429–1449.

Gabriel, Y. (2000). Storytelling in organisations: Facts, fictions and fantasies. Oxford: Oxford University Press.

Greenhalgh, T., Robert, G., Bate, P., Kyriakidou., O., Macfarlane, F., and Peacock, R. (2004). *How to Spread Good Ideas: A Systematic Review of the Literature on Diffusion, Dissemination and Sustainability of Innovations in Health Service Delivery and Organization*. London: National Coordinating Centre for the Service Delivery and Organisation R&D (NCCSDO), from http://www.sdo.lshtm.ac.uk.

Hall, G.E. and Hord, S.M. (1987). *Change in Schools*. Albany, NY: State University of New York Press.

Haynes, R.B., Devereaux, P.J., and Gyatt, G.H. (2002). Clinical expertise in the era of evidence based medicine and patient choice. *ACP Journal Club*, 136: A11–14.

Innvaer, S., Vist, G., Trommald, M., and Oxman, A. (2002). Health policy-makers' perceptions of their use of evidence: A systematic review. *Journal of Health Services & Research Policy*, 7(4): 239–244.

Kitson, A. (2004). The state of the art and science of evidence-based nursing in the UK and Europe. *Worldviews on Evidence-based Nursing*, 1: 6–8.

Locock, L., Chambers, D., Surender, R., Dopson, S., and Gabbay, J. (2001). Understanding the role of opinion leaders in improving clinical effectiveness. *Social Sciences and Medicine*, 53: 745–757.

MacDonald, G. (2002). Communication theory and health promotion. In Bunton, R. and MacDonald, G. (eds), *Health Promotion: Disciplines, Diversity and Development*. London: Rutledge.

MacGuire, W. (1978). *Evaluating Advertising: A Bibliography of the Communications Process*. New York: Advertising Research Foundations.

Michel, Y. and Sneed, N.V. (1995). Dissemination and use of research findings in nursing practice. *Journal of Professional Nursing*, 11(5), 306–311.

O'Connor, A.M., Rostom, A., Fiset, V., Tetroe, J., Entwistle, V., Llewellyn-Thomas, H.A., Holmes-Rovner, M., Barry, M., and Jones, J. (1999). Decision aids for patients facing health treatment or screening decisions: Systematic review. *British Medical Journal*, 319(7212), 731–734.

Ovretveit, J. Bate, P., Cretin, S., Gustofson, D., McInnes, K. McLeod, H., *et al.* (2002). Quality collaboratives: Lessons from research. *Quality and Safety in Health Care*, 11: 345–351.

Pierce, P.F. and Hicks, F. D. (2001). Patient decision-making behavior: An emerging paradigm for nursing science. *Nursing Research*, 50(5), 267–274.

Plsek, P.E. and Greenhalgh, T. (2001). Complexity science: The challenge of complexity in health care. *British Medical Journal*, 323: 625–628.

Reilly, B.M. (2004). The essence of EBM. *British Medical Journal*, 329: 991–992.

Rodgers, S.E. (2000). A study of the utilization of research in practice and the influence of education. *Nurse Education Today*, 20(4), 273–278.

Rogers, E. (1995). *Diffusion of Innovations*. New York: The Free Press.

Ryan (1969). *Social and Cultural Change*. New York: The Ronald Press.

Ryan, B. and Gross, N. (1943). The diffusion of hybrid seed corn in two Iowa communities. *Rural Sociology*, 8: 15–24.

Rycroft-Malone, J. (2006). The politics of evidence-based practice: Legacies and current challenges. *Journal of Research in Nursing*, 11(1), 95–108.

Rycroft-Malone J., Kitson, A., Harvey, G., McCormack, B., Seers, K., Titchen, A., and Estabrooks, C. (2002). Ingredients for change: Revisiting a conceptual framework. *Quality and Safety in Health Care*, 11: 174–180.

Sackett, D.L., Rosenberg, W.M.C., Gray, J.A.M., Haynes, R.B., and Richardson, W.S. (1996). Evidence based medicine: What it is and what it isn't (editorial). *British Medical Journal*, 312: 71–72.

Sackett, D.L., Straus, S.E., Richardson, W.S., Rosenberg, W.M.C., and Haynes, R.B. (2000). *Evidence Based Medicine: How to Practice and Teach EBM*. London: Churchill Livingston.

Sigma Theta Tau International 2005–2007 Research & Scholarship Advisory Committee. (2008). Sigma Theta Tau International Position Statement on evidence-based practice February 2007 summary. *Worldviews on Evidence-Based Nursing*, 5(2), 57–59.

Stetler, C. and Marram, G. (1976). Evaluating research findings for applicability in practice. Nursing Outlook, 24, 559–563.

Trinder, L. and Reynolds, S. (2000). *Evidence Based Practice: A Critical Appraisal*. Oxford: Blackwell Science.

Valente, T.W. (1996). Social network threshold in the diffusion of innovations. *Social Networks*, 18: 69–89.

Wejnert, B. (2002). Integrating models of diffusion of innovations: A conceptual framework. *Annual Review of Sociology*, 28: 297–326.

Wensing, M, Elwyn, G., and Grol, R. (2005). Patient-mediated strategies. In Grol, R., Wensing, M., and Eccles, M. (eds), *Improving Patient Care. The Implementation of Change in Clinical Practice*. London: Butterworth-Heinemann Elsevier.

West, E., Barron, D.N., Dowsett, J., and Newton, J.N. (1999). Hierarchies and cliques in the social networks of health care professionals: Implications for the design of dissemination strategies. *Social Science and Medicine*, 48: 633–646.

Yetton, P., Sharma, R., and Southon, G. (1999). Successful IS innovation: The contingent contributions of innovation characteristics and implementation process. *Journal of Information Technology*, 14: 53–68.

Chapter 2

Theory, frameworks, and models

Laying down the groundwork

Jo Rycroft-Malone and Tracey Bucknall

Introduction

This chapter lays down the groundwork for the remainder of the book by considering the use of theory, frameworks, and models in the pursuit of evidence-based practice (EBP). As the chapters in this book demonstrate, models and frameworks for EBP have been available for years, and in fact in some cases, decades. However, recently there has been a revived interest in the use of theory, and theoretical or conceptual frameworks as heuristics to guide EBP efforts (see Rycroft-Malone, 2007 for a fuller consideration). Perhaps it is unsurprising that there has been this renewed focus on the contribution that theory can make to our understanding of implementing EBP. Despite much financial investment over the last decade or so in pushing out evidence through tools such as clinical guidelines, and on developing the skills and knowledge of individual practitioners to appraise research, the results of these activities has been patchy. There are still large gaps between what we know and what we practice.

Theory informed evidence-based practice

In the context of EBP, research use and knowledge translation (KT), theory use and development has been presented as a promising way to better understand the "black box" of implementation; that is, what happens when individuals try and use evidence in their practice. This is based on the premise that if we can understand more about what is going on, we will be able to do things better in the future. Additionally theory is being used to guide the development of implementation interventions. Frameworks and models provide useful frames of reference to point their users in the direction of what they need to think about and pay attention to while implementing EBP.

As this begins to show, theory can be relevant to implementing EBP in a number of ways, which include:

- *Theory-based intervention development.* Often attempts to implement EBP change results in partial success or being unsuccessful. Developing KT interventions based on theory or theories has the potential to enable the development of testable theories, provide a clarity of focus (e.g., in the use of the tools one might use), facilitate explanation of findings (e.g., what works, for whom, and why), and enable the generation of theoretically transferable knowledge. Using theory provides an a priori opportunity to design an approach and/or intervention with an evidence base to believe "this might work."
- *Using theory to help identify appropriate outcomes, measures, and variables of interest.* As highlighted above, using theory provides a focus. Choosing theoretically sensitive outcomes should facilitate intervention testing, and theory development. Using theory to help the selection of measures, tools, and variables of interest, again, should facilitate appropriate evaluation, and an assessment of fit with the initial and other theories.
- *Theory-guided evaluation of implementation processes.* Developing theory inductively or applying theory more deductively could be helpful in better understanding the processes of implementing EBP. For example, there has been an increasing interest in the influence of context as a potential mediator of the use of evidence in practice. Developing theories about the mechanisms by which context could be influential may help the development of context-specific interventions. Equally, applying organizational theories to evaluations of implementation activity, may facilitate more nuanced understandings of the role that context may play.

So, the use of theory has a number of potentially useful functions for EBP, however often the theoretical underpinnings of implementation are not paid attention to (Grimshaw *et al.*, 2004). For Eccles *et al.* (2005) the case for theory use is made based on their view that previous implementation research has been "an expensive version of trial and error" (p. 108).

Often there is a lack of consistency about the way the terms theory, frameworks, and models are used, and sometimes it is not clear whether the terms are actually being used synonymously. Therefore, it is worth considering how we are using these terms, and more generally how they might be applied to implementing EBP (see Box 2.1).

What do we mean by theory?

Like most things, what we mean by theory and subsequently what we think the purpose of theory is depends on your world view. In a broad sense a theory is made up of concepts that characterize a particular phenomenon. Specifically, theory has been defined as a "way of seeing through a set of relatively concrete and specific concepts and propositions that describe or link those concepts" (after Fawcett, 1999, in Fawcett *et al.*, 2001: 117). Concepts are mental images of phenomena and propositions are statements about the concepts (Fawcett, 1999). Concepts then are the building blocks of theory. From a sociological perspective a theory is a body of related ideas that form the basis of conceptual work, and describe more than a set of phenomena; it should also explain how they work.

Box 2.1 Theory, framework, and model

A *theory* is made up of concepts that characterize a particular phenomenon. Concepts are mental images of phenomena and propositions are statements about the concepts.

A *conceptual framework* (sometimes called conceptual model) are made up of sets of concepts and the propositions that integrate them into meaningful propositions.

A *model* is narrower in scope and more precise than a conceptual framework. The concepts within a model should be well defined, and the relationships between them specific. Models are representations of the real thing; they attempt to objectify the concept they represent.

A theory can be implicit or explicit. Some explicit theories (e.g., theory of planned behavior) will be described in this, and other chapters. In contrast implicit theories are *personal* constructs about particular phenomenon; they are one's own way of knowing and thinking. The ICEBeRG group (2006) suggest that the use of explicit is more favorable than the use of implicit theory because it provides a more transparent base for the development and evaluation of interventions. However, we suggest that both types of theory can have a role to play in the implementation of EBP.

Theory can be used for different purposes: description, explanation, and prediction (see Box 2.2).

Descriptive theories describe the properties, characteristics, and qualities of a phenomenon. For example, Janes *et al.* (2008) developed a theory from a grounded theory study called "Figuring it Out in the Moment," which describes the process by which unregulated providers in special care units within long-term care facilities make decisions about and act on knowledge related to person-centered care.

Explanatory theories specify the causal relationships and mechanisms of a phenomenon, and in relation to other phenomena. For example, planned action theory is a set of interrelated concepts that explain the means by which planned change occurs (Graham and Tetroe, 2009). Graham *et al.* report on a review of planned action models to examine the components in each of the theories to determine commonalities. From this analysis they determined a number of components that may facilitate the KT processes.

Predictive theories should predict relationships between the dimensions or characteristics of the phenomenon through, for example,

---

Box 2.2 Purposes of theory

Descriptive – describe the properties, characteristics, and qualities of a phenomenon.

Explanatory theories specify the causal relationships and mechanisms of a phenomenon, and in relation to other phenomena.

Predictive theories should predict relationships between the dimensions or characteristics of the phenomenon through for example hypotheses or propositions.

hypotheses or propositions. For example, Francis *et al.* (2008) used the theory of planned behavior to explore the effects of a structured recall and prompting intervention to increase evidence-based diabetes care that was being evaluated within a pragmatic cluster randomized trial. Their use of the theory resulted in an explanation of the trial effects and support for their proposition: that attitudinally driven intentions are more consistently translated into action than those that are normatively driven (Box 2.2).

Theories are also described in terms of their scope (see Fawcett, 1999 for more detailed explanation). The highest or broadest theory is meta theory, which is a theory about a theory. A grand or macro theory encompasses a wide range of phenomena, is relatively broad, and lacks operational detail that makes it difficult to apply within empirical enquiry. There are commonalities between grand theory and conceptual frameworks (see description in the following section), and often people use these terms interchangeably because both are at a higher level of abstraction. Mid-range theories are more specific and less abstract. They are also the theories that you see most commonly applied in implementation work. This is likely to be because they encompass a smaller number of concepts, and are amenable to the development of relatively specific testable propositions or hypotheses.

So the utility of theory within implementation of EBP is in providing a guide for planning, intervention development, measurement/evaluation, and for facilitating theory development and transferability.

What do we mean by a conceptual framework?

Conceptual frameworks (sometimes called conceptual models) are by definition, made up of sets of concepts and the propositions that integrate them into meaningful propositions (Fawcett, 1999). A framework can provide anything from a skeletal set of variables to something as extensive as a paradigm; as such they can be fairly abstract. As they tend to be high level, they can apply to all types of individuals and groups, and a wide variety of situations.

Developed from the generalizations of empirical enquiry or insights conceptual frameworks facilitate the development of propositions – that is about the relationships between the concepts with the framework. Therefore their purpose is in providing a frame of reference, for organizing thinking, as a guide for what to focus on, and for interpretation. Conceptual frameworks are in a continual state of development as new evidence emerges which may challenge and augment their contents.

Ostrom (1999) developed a number of questions that could be used to test the robustness of a conceptual framework, and assess its usefulness. For example, in relation to the test of a framework's coherence, questions to ask include:

- Does the framework provide a coherent language for enabling the identification of elements of theories in relation to an important range of phenomena?
- Does the framework stimulate new theoretical developments?
- Does the framework enable the identification of differences and similarities between theories as well as their strengths and weaknesses?

For a test of usefulness, the following questions could be asked:

- Does the framework facilitate the development of empirical enquiry where there is no fully formulated theory?
- Does research that draws on the framework lead to new insights and better explanations?
- Can the framework be applied to different levels of analysis within research endeavors?

The utility of conceptual frameworks for the implementation of EBP is in their capability for being a heuristic for organizing implementation efforts: what you need to pay attention to, for assessing barriers and facilitators, generating propositions, developing theory-based interventions, etc. They should also facilitate a better understanding of what occurred during implementation; on reflection or post-hoc evaluation – what were the critical factors, were some more important than others, did particular propositions work and why, did the conceptual framework facilitate implementation, etc.

What do we mean by a model?

Models are more specific; they are narrower in scope and are more precise. The concepts within a model should be well defined, and the relationships between them specific. Models are representations of the real thing; they attempt to objectify the concept they represent. Often the term conceptual framework is used interchangeably with theoretical model. However, while both coexist with theory (Chinn and Kramer, 1991), a model offers a more precise representation and is more prescriptive.

For the implementation of EBP, a complex and multifaceted process, there is not a single theoretical model which represents KT. This is demonstrated by Estabrooks *et al.* (2006) who in their consideration of theory located a range of models from organizational, social sciences, research utilization (RU), and health promotion literatures, which are relevant to KT processes. These are listed in Table 2.1, but the reader should refer to their paper for more detail on their description and analysis.

Table 2.1 List of models relevant to knowledge translation (summarized from Estabrooks *et al.*, 2006: 26–27)

Literature/professional/ disciplinary base	Model
Social sciences	• Problem-solving model • Interactive model • Political model • Tactical model • Enlightenment model • Knowledge-driven model
Research utilization in nursing	• Conduct and Utilization of Research in Nursing (CURN) • Western Interstate Commission on Higher Education in Nursing (WICHEN) • Nursing Child Assessment Satellite Training (NCAST) • Stetler model (see Chapter 3 for full description of this model) • Iowa model of research use in practice (see Chapter 6 for full description of this model)
Health promotion	• Readiness to change model
Organizational	• Model of territorial rights and boundaries • Dual core model of the innovation • Ambidextrous model • Bandwagon models • Desperation reaction model

Summary

Clearly what is meant by theory, conceptual frameworks, and models is inextricably linked by core characteristics: concepts, hypotheses/ propositions, and more or less structured linkages. However, each varies in terms of their specificity and prescriptiveness. For the implementation of evidence into practice, all are heuristics that have the potential to:

- inform the development of research, development, and quality improvement questions;
- guide the choice and development of implementation interventions;
- facilitate an appropriate choice of tools and measurement devices, and variables of interest;
- direct the user toward appropriate implementation and evaluation methodology and methods;
- facilitate the development of new knowledge, insights, and theory.

The ways these devices can be applied is considered in the following sections and the remainder of this book.

Using theory and frameworks for implementing evidence-based practice

Having considered what we mean by theory, frameworks, and models, this section considers the use of these mental devises for implementing EBP. While the underlying motivation for developing this book was concerned with making theory use and development more obvious within attempts to implement evidence into practice, there are others who are more skeptical about this. These skeptics express a number of concerns (e.g., Bhattacharyya *et al.*, 2006; Oxman *et al.*, 2005), which are worth reflecting on now before our consideration about the various ways that theory could be helpful.

Broadly, those that have concerns about the recent turn to theory within the KT literature argue that (a) there is a lack of evidence to support the idea of theory use, (b) the selection of theories for use can be at best arbitrary because there are limited criteria to help us choose among them, and (c) common sense, sound logic, and rigorous evaluation should be the guiding principles that we use when designing implementation interventions. There is a further argument made by the skeptics, which builds on the consideration of the complexities of implementation. Within our first chapter we made the case for the need to acknowledge the complex, multifaceted nature of implementation processes. It has been argued that applying theory in these complex situations could be constraining because being confined to theory-driven interventions potentially neglects the interactions, key processes, and relationships. In fact, we would argue that whether you are constrained or not, depends on how you both develop and/or apply theory in implementation work. As we said earlier, it depends on the world view you take.

Positivism facilitates deterministic explanations, that is, if you do x, y is likely to happen. However, there are also other ways that theory can be used. For example, Charmaz (2006) makes the case for an interpretive approach because it emphasizes understanding rather than explanation. Rather than seeking causality and linearity (positivism), interpretative theories can be used to prioritize connections and patterns. However, to date, theory use in the implementation of EBP has tended to be more deterministic, than for example, interpretive.

The examples of theory use in the literature have tended to focus on relatively straightforward clinical issues (e.g., sore throat), change in individual's behavior (e.g., a physician's prescribing practice), and on applying single theories (e.g., theory of planned behavior) (e.g., Eccles *et al.*, 2005; Grol and Grimshaw, 2003). The application of the theory of planned behavior is now commonly used and tested as a predictive theory for determining individual behavior (change). For example, Eccles *et al.* (2009) explored the relationship between the theory of planned behavior's direct predictors of behavior (individuals' intentions and perceived behavioral control). More specifically they wanted to see if the collective intentions of individuals could predict team performance. Using two clinical behaviors: statin prescription and food examination in the management of patients with diabetes, they gathered data from a sample of primary care doctors and nurses in England and the Netherlands. Data were collected via a questionnaire survey developed from the constructs of the theory of planned behavior, and patient reported data on clinical outcomes. Findings showed that none of the aggregated scores predicted statin prescription, but the highest intention in the team was a significant predictor of foot examination. They conclude by suggesting that aggregating individually administered measures may be a methodological advance of theoretical importance.

The preceding paragraph outlines a particular illustration of theory use and application. The theory of planned behavior is an appealing psychological theory for implementing EBP. First, it is a way of explaining behavior, but also if one can predict the way that individuals might behave (e.g., make a clinical decision, prescribe certain medications, etc.) then one might be able to develop more effective behavioral interventions. However, given that there are many factors, at multiple levels (e.g., individual, team, organization) that might predict the use of evidence in practice, one can see why some might be skeptical of this type of theory use.

As the contents of this book demonstrate, there are many ways to use, apply, and develop theory, which includes inductive and deductive approaches, and a combination of both. The challenge is to design studies that not only pay attention to theory (whether that is implicit or explicit) but also facilitate an exploration beyond the parameters a theory might prescribe. Approaches such as realistic evaluation (Pawson and Tilley, 1997) place an emphasis on what, why, and how questions, which not only require the development of explanatory theoretical frameworks, but could also incorporate the application of explicit mid-range theory.

The theory menu

The menu of potentially useable explicit mid-range theory is extensive. Relevant theory for implementing EBP, comes from a wide variety of evidential and disciplinary bases including health promotion, social sciences, organizational development, marketing, decision-making science, and education (see examples in Table 2.2, Grol *et al.*, 2005, Michie *et al.*, 2005 for an in-depth consideration of explicit mid-range theory). Taking examples from these various levels of application (i.e., individual, group, organization) it is possible to see how theory can inform the implementation of EBP.

There are many relevant theories that could be applied at the level of the *individual*. Individual behavior does, to a greater or lesser extent, influence whether evidence gets used in practice. We have already outlined examples from the literature of the use of the theory of planned behavior, which assumes individual behavior is motivated, and therefore predicted by motivation. Other relevant theories come from decision-making science (see Bucknall, 2007 for an overview).

Table 2.2 Examples of relevant theories for implementation

Level	Examples of theories

Individual (relevant to practitioners and patients)	• Decision making, and cognitive theories
	  – Cognitive continuum theory
	• Educational theories
	  – Theory of transformative learning
	  – Adult learning theory
	  – Social learning theory
	• Attitudinal theories
	• Motivational theories
	  – Social cognition theory
	  – Theory of planned behavior
	• Marketing theories
	• Changes theories
	  – Transtheoretical model of change

Group	• Social network theories • Social learning theories • Communities of practice theories • Social capital theories • Communication theories • Leadership theories
Organization	• Institutional theory • Organizational culture theories • Agency theory • Change theories • Complexity theory • Economic theories • Organizational learning theory • Configuration theory • Actor-network theory • Structuration theory • Contingency theory

For example, cognitive continuum theory (Hammond, 1988) represents decision making on a continuum that has analysis at one end and intuition at the other. How individuals make decisions, that is, more or less analytical or intuitive, are determined by the characteristics of the decision. The decision can range from ill to well structured. It is hypothesized that the greater the task structure, the higher the level of analysis involved in the decision-making process, which is also influenced by time factors and complexity of available information. As Bucknall (2007) suggests, the application of this theory to implementation is in the opportunity it affords to map decision-making processes while undertaking different types of activities. It could also be used to guide the development of an intervention to improve decision making in cases where there are varying amounts of information/evidence.

Often education is used as an intervention within implementation projects. Applying educational theory to these interventions might (a) increase the chances of it being successful, and (b) help explain why or why not it was effective. For example, adult learning theory (Knowles, 1984) assumes a number of things about the adult learner, which would be helpful to pay attention to in the development of education interventions. These include that adults are self directed, they bring their own experiences and knowledge to the situation and acquire knowledge more easily if it is relevant and considered alongside their prior knowledge, and that they wish to be treated with respect. Therefore, when designing interventions applying the theory of adult learning it would be sensible to assess participants' existing knowledge, ascertain their needs, build training and education around acquiring appropriate and meaningful information, deliver sessions that build on adults' desire to be self directive, offer opportunities for interaction, and provision of feedback about learning.

At the *group* level, there are a number of mid-range theories that might be useful for application within implementation activities. These theories focus on change being a determinant of the interaction between individuals and others. For example, this could include interaction with peers, networks, opinion leaders, and patients. Relevant theories include social network and influence theory, social learning theory, and leadership theories (see Table 2.2). For example, social learning theory determines that changing practice is a function of learning by experience, and watching the behavior of others, including reinforcement of "correct" behavior. Therefore in applying social learning theory to changing behavior or improving performance/practice might include elements to help motivate change including role modeling of appropriate practice (within context) by for example, an opinion leader. It would also be important to put mechanisms in place that provide positive reinforcement for appropriate behavior. Another example of relevant theory at group level is theories about social networks. Communities of practice have become a phenomenon of interest within the KT community as a mechanism for sharing and particularizing knowledge locally through interaction. Applying social network theory to mechanisms like communities of practice would facilitate a better understanding of the characteristics of the linkages between network members, the ways that knowledge and information is transferred between them, and whether and how that knowledge is used. Additionally applying social network theory to knowledge transfer intervention development would lead to an intervention based on networks and interactions between key stakeholders.

Equally, at the level of the *organization* there are many theories that could be applied to the implementation of evidence into practice. This level of theory is particularly helpful in increasing understanding of the contextual (including cultural) factors that might affect, and be affecting successful implementation (SI). For example, the theory of learning organizations is relevant for understanding how particular types of organizations effectively and efficiently implement practice changes and innovations. Similarly theories on organizational culture have relevance to understanding conducive contexts and cultures. For example Scott *et al.* (2003) found that performance and culture is often linked. Drawing on concepts from learning organizations, in their analysis of organizational studies, they found that organizations that had formal structures and regulations, in contrast to those that had effective team working, role clarity, and good coordination, were less likely to be successful in quality improvement activity. Using organizational theories can provide a lens through which to under-stand the organizational factors that may be facilitating or hindering implementation, as well as providing some guidance as to what might need to be paid attention to at an organizational level if implementation interventions are to be successful (see Scott *et al.*, 2003, for a more in-depth consideration of these issues).

As well as theories at the individual, group, and organizational level, there are also *process theories* that could be applied in implementation projects. Graham and Tetroe (2009) suggest that a planned action theory is a set of logically interrelated concepts that explain the way that change occurs, predicts how various environmental factors will react in situations of change, and help those planning change control those variables that increase or decrease the likelihood of successful change. In this sense, planned action theories are predictive theories. They recently completed a theory analysis of 31 planned action theories (see Graham and Tetroe, 2009 for more detail). From this, they identified a number of core components of all the theories (however not all theories included each component), which results in 10 action steps.

 (1) Identify the problem that needs addressing
 (2) Review the literature
 (3) Adapt the evidence/literature and/or develop the innovation
 (4) Assess the barriers to using the knowledge
 (5) Select and tailor interventions to promote the use of the evidence
 (6) Implement the innovation
 (7) Develop a plan to evaluate use of the knowledge
 (8) Evaluate the impact or outcomes of the innovation
 (9) Maintain change and sustain ongoing knowledge use
(10) Disseminate results of the implementation processes.

Their suggestion is that before choosing a particular planned action theory, it is important to assess which of the above components are present, to ascertain whether the particular theory would be fit for purpose. From their analysis Graham and Tetroe developed the Knowledge To Action (KTA) framework, which is described in more detail in Chapter 10.

Choosing theory

As there are many theories to choose from – choosing appropriate theory is a potential challenge. A number of criteria have been proposed that could facilitate this choice including whether the theory is robust, logical, generalizable, testable, useful, and appropriate (Eccles *et al.*, 2005; ICEBeRG, 2006; Rycroft-Malone, 2007) (see Box 2.3 for more details).

In reality, applying these criteria will only reduce the extensive list, not necessarily identify the "ideal" theory. Additionally, implementing complex interventions will likely mean that it is necessary to consider the application of more than one theory, so the appropriate choice of a suite of theories will likely be required. One suggestion in cases such as this would be to use an overarching theoretical framework, which could be populated by relevant mid-range theories. An illustration of this was provided by Rycroft-Malone (2007) through the application of the Promoting Action on Research Implementation in Health Services (PARIHS) framework (see Chapter 5 for a description of PARIHS). The hypothesis offered by the PARIHS framework is that SI is a function of the nature and perceptions of the *evidence*, the quality of the *context*, and the way in which the process is *facilitated*. It was suggested that in applying the PARIHS framework

Box 2.3 Choosing between theories: some criteria and questions

What are the origins of the theory?

This refers to how the theory was developed. Key questions to ask are: Who developed it? Was the theory developed within a particular discipline? How was the theory developed? Is there evidence to support or refute the theory?

What is the meaning of the theory?

This question refers to the concepts that make up the theory. Key questions to ask are: What concepts make up the theory? Are these well described? Is it clear how the concepts relate to each other?

Is the theory logically consistent?

This criterion refers to the internal consistency of the theory. Therefore key questions to ask are: Are the concepts within the theory logically connected? Are the statements and propositions coherent and logical?

Is the theory parsimonious and generalizable?

Key questions to ask for this criterion include: Is the theory simple but still able to encapsulate the phenomenon? Does the theory have the potential to enable generalization?

Is the theory useful?

Using theory needs to be a helpful undertaking, therefore being able to say "yes" to question such as "is the theory going to help me understand more about this issue"? or "is the theory going to be helpful in the development of this intervention"? is critical.

Is the theory testable?

For theory to be useful it needs to be testable. Therefore key questions to ask of the theory are: does the theory enable the generation of testable hypotheses and/or propositions? Is the theory supported by empirical data? Can the theory be used within different methodological approaches?

Is the theory appropriate?

It is important that the theory chosen is fit for purpose, therefore questions to ask include: is this theory appropriate for the target group? Is this theory relevant to this particular situation, including context, and implementation topic?

After ICEBeRG (2006) and Rycroft-Malone (2007).

a number of mid-range theories could be considered relevant to a study aiming at improving outcomes while evaluating how and why interventions worked or not:

- Dual processing models of reasoning (e.g., Sladek *et al.*, 2006), which would help identify and explain individual differences in the way practitioners moderated their decisions to incorporate new *evidence*.
- Structuration theory (e.g., Giddens, 1984), which would be helpful in discovering the links between *context* ("structure") and action (in this case behavior of practitioners in incorporating evidence into practice), and in understanding the dynamic processes between context and action.
- Adult learning theory (Knowles, 1984), which facilitators use as part of a *facilitation* intervention could be tested alongside the application of, for example, social influence theory (Mittman *et al.*, 1992).

This is just one example of how a conceptual framework can be used as a container or heuristic for the consideration of different theories and theoretical perspectives. Additionally, using conceptual frameworks could enable the development of inductive theory (see the following section).

Why a theory might not work

While theory is likely to be helpful (to a greater or lesser extent) in developing implementation interventions, as the ICEBeRG group (2006) point out, there are reasons why the use of explicit theory might not work. The reasons they offer include:

(1) The theory itself might be "faulty" or inadequate. If a theory has been poorly defined (e.g., concepts lack clarity) and/or inadequately described, its application within intervention development is likely to work in a predicable way.
(2) The choice of theory might not be appropriate to the particular circumstances or context of the implementation activity. For example, there is little point applying a theory that relates to individual practitioner behavior if an organizational level intervention is required. The ICEBeRG group suggest that in such situations rather than using a less than ideal mid-range theory, one should consider the use of implicit or practice level theory.

(3) The theory-based intervention itself is not well operationalized. This could lead to a lack of clarity about the actual effect of the intervention, and potentially result in diverting attention away from the factors that are in fact influencing outcomes.

Therefore if theory is to be of use, careful consideration is required when developing project ideas, intervention development and testing, and also in monitoring progress. If theory use is "faulty," ultimately it is not going to be helpful for implementing evidence into practice.

Models and frameworks

Just as there are many theories that are available and relevant to the implementation of EBP, there are also many conceptual and theoretical frameworks and models. Sudsawad (2007) published a selective review of KT models and frameworks and categorized them as: Interaction-focused frameworks; Context-focused models and frameworks; and Individual-focused models. Table 2.3 lists the frameworks included within these categories.

As the table shows, some of these models and frameworks are described in more detail in this book. It was not Sudsawad's intention to provide a comprehensive review, and indeed there are many other models and frameworks that could have been included in her list. We, too, do not provide a comprehensive text on all the available frameworks and models that could be useful in the implementation of EBP. Therefore readers may also be interested in the following frameworks and models and consider their potential utility for implementation. The criteria we used to analyze the frameworks and models in this book (see Tables 2.4 and 2.5) could provide a useful tool or checklist to help determine a framework or model's suitability or fit for purpose.

- Greenhalgh *et al.* (2004a, b) developed a "conceptual model" from an evidence synthesis of the diffusions of innovations, quality improvement, and diffusions of innovation theoretical and empirical literature. Their framework has a number of components including: system antecedents for change (e.g., structure, absorptive capacity, receptive context); system readiness (e.g., resources, tension for change); adopter (needs, motivation, values and goals, skills, learning style, and social networks); assimilation (complex,

Table 2.3 Models and frameworks included in Sudsawad's review

Category	Model or framework
Interaction-focused frameworks	Understanding user-context framework (Jacobson *et al.*, 2003). A framework for increasing the potential of user involvement in the knowledge translation process.
Context-focused models and frameworks	The Ottawa Model of Research Use (Graham and Logan, 2004) (see Chapter 4 in this book)
	The Knowledge To Action process framework (Graham *et al.*, 2006) (see Chapter 10 in this book)
	The Promoting Action on Research Implementation in Health Services (PARIHS) framework (Kitson *et al.*, 1998; Rycroft-Malone *et al.*, 2002) (see Chapter 5 in this book)
	The coordinated implementation model (Lomas, 1993). This model represents the environmental factors that might influence the research implementation process.
Individual-focused models	The Stetler model of research utilization (Stetler, 2001) (see Chapter 3 in this book)

nonlinear); implementation process (e.g., decision-making, dedicated resources, feedback on process); linkage (e.g., shared meaning, effective knowledge transfer, communication, and information); outer context (e.g., incentives and mandates, environmental stability); communication and influence (from diffusion to dissemination); and innovation (e.g., relative advantage, trialability, risk, nature of knowledge). The authors suggest that the model could be used as an aide memoir for considering the different aspects of the complexity of innovation adoption.

- The Conduct and Utilization of Research in Nursing (CURN) is one of the oldest models of RU (Horsley *et al.*, 1978). Developed inductively from the findings from a large multisite (*n* = 31) project conducted in Michigan in the USA, the goal of this model is to guide practice change. The model is problem focused and takes an organizational perspective to changing practice. For example, assumptions include that the organization is committed to the process, and that there are available and substantive resources

Table 2.4 Criteria for assessing model and framework development

	Type		Purpose			Development		Theoretical underpinning		Conceptual clarity
	Model	Framework	Descriptive	Explanatory	Predictive	Inductive	Deductive	Implicit	Explicit	
Model										

Table 2.5 Criteria for assessing model and framework application

Models	Levels				Situation			Users					Function				Testable
	Individual	Team	Unit	Organization	Policy	Hypothetical	Real	Nurses	Medics	Allied health	Multidisciplinary	Policy makers	Assessment of facilitators and barriers	Intervention/strategy development	Outcome measurement and variable selection	Evaluation of process	

dedicated to it. The CURN model is a planned action theory, and as such it contains a number of process steps:

(1) systematic identification of a problem
(2) identification of an evidence/literature base
(3) transformation of the evidence into a solution or protocol
(4) clinical trial or other evaluation
(5) decision
(6) development of an approach to extending or diffusing a new practice
(7) development of mechanisms to sustain practice changes over time.

- Grol and Wensing (2004) have also developed a planned action theory model, which includes a number of steps or processes; the sequence of which they state may depend on different situations and circumstances. The steps are similar to those of other planned action theories including the identification of a problem; the development of a concrete proposal; analysis of performance, development/selection of strategies; and measures to change practice, development, testing; and execution of implementation plan, and continuous evaluation and adaptation (where necessary).

- May *et al.* (2007) have developed The Normalization Process Model, which they describe as a theoretical model that can be used to explain how complex interventions become embedded in practice. Developed from the analysis of empirical studies it contains four factors, which inhibit or facilitate normalization: interactional workability, relational integration, skill set workability, and contextual integration. They suggest that the model could be used as applied theory to develop hypotheses about the outcomes of normalization processes. Additionally as a theoretical framework May *et al.* propose that it can help identify and describe factors that facilitate or inhibit the implementation of complex interventions, and that it could be used for identifying the probability that complex interventions might become routinely embedded in practice.

In addition to these specific examples of models and frameworks, interaction approaches are also gaining prominence. At a local level, there is a growing evidence base to suggest that a "sensemaking" process takes place that influences how research is enacted in clinical practice. This in turn is influenced by local context and background organizational capacity (e.g., Dopson and Fitzgerald, 2005). Therefore knowledge use and exchange can be conceptualized as an interaction between research users and producers. In the literature these approaches are called different things including integrated KT, mode 2 research, and interactive research. Such approaches are gaining prominence because they acknowledge the messy, complex, social, and dynamic nature of knowledge use. However, their role in more proactive implementation efforts has yet to be articulated. The premise that collaboration and partnerships between the producers and users of research might increase knowledge uptake makes sense. These ideas have yet to be fully tested.

Models and frameworks included in this book

To help our choice of which frameworks and models to include in this book we developed some criteria and sought the opinion of a number of experts in the field. The criteria we used included:

(1) Models/frameworks should be recognized internationally; that is they have been published in international journals and are cited in international literature by others.
(2) The models/frameworks have been subject to evaluation and/or testing (not just by the authors).
(3) That the models/frameworks are transferable across different settings (i.e., hospitals, clinical contexts), regions, and countries.
(4) That we include a sample of models/frameworks from across disciplines.
(5) That the models/frameworks we include represent a range from those that are well established to those that are newer to the literature.
(6) Those that have been involved in the development of the models/ framework were willing to author the chapter and use a standard template to enable cross model/framework synthesis.

These criteria resulted in the following models/frameworks being included:

- Stetler model
- Ottawa Model of Research Use (OMRU)
- Promoting Action on Research Implementation in Health Services (PARIHS) framework
- Iowa model of evidence-based practice

- Advancing Research and Clinical practice through close Collaboration (ARCC) model
- Dobbins' dissemination and use of research evidence for policy and practice framework
- Joanna Briggs Institute model
- Knowledge To Action framework

Approach to analysis and synthesis

In order to facilitate our analysis and synthesis of the models and frameworks in the proceeding chapters we developed a framework (see Tables 2.4 and 2.5). The subject areas for the framework were developed from the content of this chapter, particularly in relation to choosing theory and assessing the robustness and usefulness of frameworks. The following sections describe how we interpreted and therefore applied each domain in our assessment of each model and/or framework.

Model or framework?

- A framework can provide anything from a skeletal set of variables to something as extensive as a paradigm; as such they can be fairly abstract.
- A model is a more precise representation and is more prescriptive.

Purpose?

- *Descriptive:* The framework or model describes the properties, characteristics, and qualities of a phenomenon.
- *Explanatory:* The framework or model specifies causal relationships and mechanisms of a phenomenon, and in relation to other phenomena.
- *Predictive:* The framework or model predicts relationships between the dimensions or characteristics of the phenomenon through for example hypotheses or propositions.

Development

- Was the framework/model developed inductively or deductively?
- Was the framework/model developed from empirical and/or collective insights?
- Is there evidence to support or refute the framework/model?

Theoretical underpinnings

Are the theoretical underpinnings of the framework or model explicit, or are they implicit?

Conceptual clarity

- Does the framework or model have a well described and coherent language for enabling the identification of key elements?
- Does the framework or model enable the identification of similarities and differences between theories as well as their strengths and weaknesses?
- Does the framework or model have the potential to stimulate new theoretical developments?

Levels

Is the framework or model applicable at an individual, team, unit, organization, and/or policy level?

Situation

Could the framework or model be used in hypothetical (e.g., classroom, simulation) and/or real situations?

Users

Who are the relevant or intended users of the framework or model? (i.e., Nurses/medics/allied health/multidisciplinary/policy makers)

Function

Can the framework or model be used for:

- Assessment of facilitators and barriers
- Intervention development
- Outcome measurement and variable selection
- Evaluation of processes

Testable

- Does the framework or model enable the generation of testable hypotheses and/or propositions?
- Is the framework or model supported by empirical data?
- Could the framework or model be used within different methodological approaches?

Contributors to the book were asked to describe their framework or model using predetermined headings, which facilitated the application of the above criteria. Each chapter was read by the editors and a judgment made about how each model or framework met the criteria. These judgments were then developed into a narrative synthesis; our analysis and the synthesis are presented in Chapter 11.

Summary

This chapter has set the context for the remainder of the book. It has described some core concepts in relation to theory, frameworks, and models and linked these to the implementation of evidence into practice. Explicit theory and frameworks can be used in different ways including intervention development, identification of appropriate outcomes, measures and variables of interest, and for theory-guided evaluation of implementation processes. Equally, there is a place for implicit theory application and development, particularly in cases where there is not an appropriate mid-range theory or robust framework or model available for use. There is a large menu of mid-range theories and many frameworks and models available for use in the implementation of EBP, therefore we have developed some criteria for readers to use to help them identify which of those might be appropriate or fit for purpose. The following chapters describe a number of different frameworks and models for the implementation of evidence into practice. These have been ordered chronologically, that is, from those that are older to those that are newer. Their key features and potential applications are then synthesized in Chapter 11.

References

Bhattacharyya, O., Reeves, S., Garfinkel, S., and Zwarenstein, M. (2006). Designing theoretically informed implementation interventions: Fine in theory, but evidence of effectiveness in practice is needed. *Implementation Science*, 1, 5. Available at: http://www.implementationscience.com/content/1/1/5

Bucknall, T. (2007). A gaze through the lens of decision theory toward knowledge translation science. *Nursing Research*, 56(4S), S60–S65.

Charmaz, K. (2006). *Constructing grounded theory: A practical guide through qualitative analysis*. London, Sage.

Chinn, P.L. and Kramer, M.K. (1991). *Theory and nursing* (3rd edn). St. Louis, Mosby-Year Book, Inc.

Dopson, S and Fitzgerald, L. (eds). (2005). *Knowledge to action? Evidence-based health care in context*. Oxford, Oxford University Press.

Eccles, M., Grimshaw, J., Walker, A., Johnston, M., and Pitts, N. (2005). Changing the behaviour of healthcare professionals: The use of theory in promoting the uptake of research findings. *Journal of Clinical Epidemiology*, 58, 107–112.

Eccles, M., Hrisos, S., Francis, J.J., Steen, N., Bosch, M., and Johnston, M. (2009). Can the collective intentions of individual professionals within healthcare teams predict the team's performance: Developing methods and theory. *Implementation Science*. Available at: http://www.implementationscience.com/content/4/1/24

Estabrooks, C.A., Thompson, D.S., Lovely, J.E., and Hofmeyer, A. (2006). A guide to knowledge translation theory. *The Journal of Continuing Education in the Health Professions*, 26, 25–36.

Fawcett, J. (1999). *The relationship of theory and research* (3rd edn). Philadelphia, FA Davies.

Fawcett, J., Watson, J., Neuman, B., Walker, P.H., and Fitzpatrick, J.J. (2001). On nursing theories and evidence. *Journal of Nursing Scholarship*, 33(2), 115–119.

Francis, J.J., Eccles, M., Johnson, M., Whitty, P., Grimshaw, J.M., Kaner, E.F.S., Smith, L., and Walker, A. (2008). Explaining the effects of an intervention designed to promote evidence-based diabetes care: A theory-based process evaluation of a pragmatic cluster randomised controlled trial. *Implementation Science*, 3, 50. Available at: http://www.implementationsciences.com/content/3/1/50

Giddens, A. (1984). *The constitution of society: Outline of the theory of structuration*. Cambridge, Polity.

Graham, I. and Logan, J. (2004). Innovations in knowledge transfer and continuity of care. *Canadian Journal of Nursing Research*, 36, 89–103.

Graham, I.D., Logan, J., Harrison, M.B., Straus, S., Tetroe, J., and Caswell, W. (2006). Lost in knowledge translation: Time for a map? *The Journal of Continuing Education in the Health Professions*, 26, 13–24.

Graham, I. and Tetroe, J. (2009). Planned action theories. In: Straus, S., Tetroe, J., and Graham, I. (eds), *Knowledge translation in health care*. Oxford, Wiley Blackwell and BMJ Books, pp. 185–195.

Greenhalgh, T., Robert, G., Bate, P., Kyriakidou, O., Macfarlane, F., and Peacock, R. (2004a). *How to spread good ideas. A systematic review of the literature on diffusion, dissemination and sustainability of innovations in health service delivery and organisation*. London, National Co-ordinating Centre for NHS Service Delivery and Organisation. Available at: http://www.sdo.lshtm.ac.uk.

Greenhalgh, T., Robert, G., Macfarlane, F., Bate, P., and Kyriakidou, O. (2004b). Diffusion of innovations in service organizations: Systematic review and recommendations. *Milbank Quarterly*, 82(4), 581–629.

Grimshaw, J.M., Thomas, R.E., MacLennan, G., Fraser, C., Ramsay, C.R., Vale, L., *et al.* (2004). Effectiveness and efficiency of guideline dissemination and implementation strategies. *Health Technology Assessment*, 8, 1–72.

Grol, R. and Grimshaw, J.M. (2003). From best evidence to best practice: Effective implementation of change to patients' care. *Lancet*, 362, 1225–1230.

Grol, R. and Wensing, M. (2004). What drives change? Barriers to and incentives for achieving evidence-based practice. *MJA*, 180, S57–S60.

Grol, R., Wensing, M., and Eccles, M. (2005). *Improving patient care. The implementation of change in clinical practice*. London, Elsevier.

Hammond, K.R. (1988). Clinical intuition and clinical analysis: Expertise and the cognitive continuum. In: Dowie, J. and Elstein, A. (eds), *Professional judgement: A reader in clinical decision making*. Cambridge, Cambridge University Press.

Horsley, J.A., Crane, J., and Bingle, J.D. (1978). Research utilization as an organizational process. *Journal of Nursing Administration*, 8, 4–6.

ICEBeRG Group. (2006). Designing theoretically informed implementation interventions. *Implementation Science*, 1, 4. Available at: http://www.implementationscience/com/content/1/1/4

Jacobson, N., Butterill, D., and Goering, P. (2003). Development of a framework for knowledge translation: Understanding user context. *Journal of Health Services Research & Policy*, 8, 94–99.

Janes, N., Souraya, S., Cott, C., Rappolt, S., and Reg, O.T. (2008). Figuring it Out in the Moment: A theory of unregulated care providers' knowledge utilization in dementia care. *Worldviews on Evidence-Based Nursing*, 5(1), 13–24.

Kitson, A.L., Harvey, G., and McCormack, B. (1998). Enabling the implementation of evidence-based practice: A conceptual framework. *Quality in Health Care*, 7(3), 149–158.

Knowles, M.S. (1984). *Andragogy in action*. San Franscisco, Jossey Bass.

Lomas, J. (1993). Retailing research: Increasing the role of evidence in clinical services for childbirth. *Milbank Quarterly*, 71, 439–475.

May, C., Finch, T., Mair, F., Ballini, L., Dowrick, C., Eccles, M., Gask, L., MacFarlane, A., Murray, E., Rapley, T., Rogers, A., Treweek, S., Wallace, P., Anderson, B.J., and Heaven, B. (2007). Understanding the implementation of complex interventions in health care: The normalization process model. *Implementation Science*, 7, 148. Available at: http://www.biomedcentral.com/1472-6963/7/148 last accessed 1 March 2009.

Michie, S., Johnston, M., Abraham, C., Lawton, R., Parker, D., and Walker, A. (2005). Making psychological theory useful for implementing evidence-based practice: A consensus approach. *Quality and Safety in Health Care*, 14, 26–33.

Mittman, B.S., Tonesk, X., and Jacobson, P.D. (1992). Implementing clinical practice guidelines: Social influence strategies and practitioner behaviour change. *Qualitative Review Bulletin*, 18, 413–422.

Ostrom, E. (1999). Institutional rational choice: An assessment of the institutional analysis and development framework. In: Sabatier, P.A. (ed.), *Theories of the policy press.* Colorado, Westview Press.

Oxman, A.D., Fretheim, A., and Flottrop, S. (2005). The OFF theory of research utilization. *Journal of Clinical Epidemiology*, 58, 113–116.

Pawson, R. and Tilley, N. (1997). *Realist evaluation.* London, Sage Publications.

Rycroft-Malone, J. (2007). Theory and knowledge translation: Setting some co-ordinates? *Nursing Research*, 56(4S), S78–S85.

Rycroft-Malone, J., Kitson, A., Harvey, G., McCormack, B., Seers, K., Titchen, A., and Estabrooks, C.A. (2002). Ingredients for change: Revisiting a conceptual framework. *Quality and Safety in Health Care*, 11, 174–180.

Scott, T., Mannion, R., Davies, H., and Marshall, M. (2003). Healthcare performance and organisational culture. Oxford, Radcliffe Medical Press.

Sladek, R.M., Phillips, A., xand Bond, M.J. (2006). Implementation science: A role for parallel dual processing models of reasoning? *Implementation Science*, 1, 12. Available at: http://www.implementation science/com/content/1/12

Stetler, S. (2001). Updating the Stetler model of research utilization to facilitate evidence-based practice. *Nursing Outlook*, 49, 272–278.

Sudsawad, P. (2007). *Knowledge translation. Introduction to models, strategies and measures.* Austin, TX, Southwest Education Development Laboratory, The National Center for the Dissemination of Disability Research. Available at: http://www.ncddr.org/kt/products/ktintro/ktintro. pdf (last accessed 1 July 2009).

Chapter 3

Stetler model

Cheryl B. Stetler

Key learning points

- A prescriptive, critical thinking model consisting of interactive, criteria-based decision-making steps, that is, this model makes the process of decision making regarding use of evidence explicit and transparent for the user.
- Initially, an individual-level or "practitioner"-focused model; currently useful for both individuals and groups making a collective decision.
- An evidence-based practice model with a primary focus on research evidence implementation, but with clear consideration of supplemental forms of evidence.
- Evolved over decades of use into a package of published resources and tools.

Introduction and purpose of the model

In the 1970s, the conduct of nursing research and its role in the profession was an international topic of discussion in the literature (Birch, 1979; Bloch, 1979; Harrison, 1978). Articles were published regarding use or the need to use research in practice (Diers, 1972; Gunter, 1971). However, in the early to mid-1970s, little in the way of guidance was available for those wishing to teach students or staff nurses how to actually go about using research. The majority of nursing research texts at the time offered little direction for the implementation of evidence into practice. Thus, the initial form of the Stetler model was developed (Stetler and Marram, 1976).

The Stetler model is a prescriptive, *critical thinking* approach. It consists of a sequence of interactive, criterion-based *decision-making steps* designed to facilitate effective use of research and other relevant evidence. As a "planned action theory", it is a conceptual model that outlines "steps to deliberately engineer change" (Graham and Tetroe, 2009). The model's purpose is to provide guidance for the careful "thinking through" or problem-solving process of determining (a) the applicability of research and additional evidence to a specific practice-related issue; (b) the exact nature of the evidence to be applied and implications for its conversion into a useable form; and (c) the how-to's of effective implementation and evaluation of acceptable evidence in practice. The model has long been considered a *practitioner-oriented* model (Kim, 1999; Stetler and Marram, 1976). However, the model applies not only to the use of evidence by a knowledgeable, individual practitioner; it also applies to groups of practitioners on a committee or project team. Although the term practitioner often implies bedside clinicians, in this model, "practice" additionally relates to the activities of administrators, managers, educators, and other health care specialists.

The two-part 2009 Stetler model of evidence-based practice (EBP) is presented in Fig. 3.1A, B. It highlights critical phases, concepts, and decisions that must be made if use is to be safe, appropriate, feasible, and effective for individual practitioners and EBP groups. Its primary focus, as in other models of EBP, is the *use of research*; however, *supplemental use of other forms of evidence* is also recognized. Definitions now integral to the model are as follows (Ciliska *et al.*, 2005; Rycroft-Malone and Stetler, 2004; Stetler *et al.*, 1998a; Stetler, 2001a):

- *Evidence-based practice*: A problem-solving approach to professional practice that bases relevant decisions and practice strategies on the best available evidence.
- *Evidence*: Credible, verifiable data, facts, or information that have been systematically obtained.
- *Affirmed experience*: Experiences that are externalized for purposes of reflection, verification, and evaluation; affirmed experience is contrasted with unsystematic clinical experience, including "experiential" opinions based on isolated events, potentially incomplete or inaccurate observations, or perceptions that are not validated.

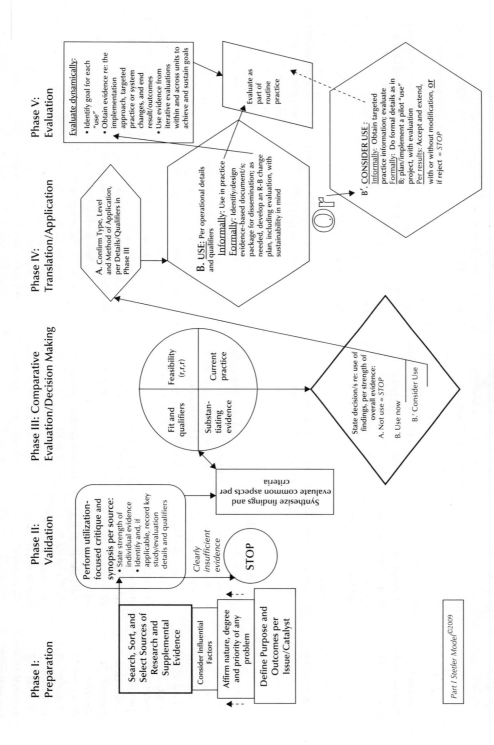

Phase I: Preparation

Phase II: Validation

Phase III: Comparative Evaluation/Decision Making

Phase IV: Translation/Application

Phase V: Evaluation

Figure 3.1 Stetler Model of evidence-based practice © 2009 Cheryl Stetler

Part I Stetler Model©2009

Phase I: Preparation	Phase II: Validation	Phase III: Comparative Evaluation/Decision Making	Phase IV: Translation/Application	Phase V: Evaluation
Purpose, Context, & Sources of Evidence:	Credibility of Evidence & Potential for/ Detailed Qualifiers of Application:	Synthesis & Decisions/ Recommendations per Criteria of Applicability:	Operational Definition of Use/Actions for Change:	Alternative Evaluations:
• **Potential Issues/Catalysts** = a problem, including *unexplained variations; less-than-best practice; routine update of knowledge; validation/ routine revision of procedures, etc; or innovative program goal*	• **Critique & synopsize essential components, operational details, and other qualifying factors, per source** • *See instructions for use of utilization-focused review tables;* with *evaluative criteria, to facilitate this task; fill in the tables for group decision making or potential future synthesis*	• ***Synthesize the cumulative findings:** • *Logically organize & display the similarities and differences across multiple findings, per common aspects or sub-elements of the topic under review* • *Evaluate degree of substantiation of each aspect/sub-element; reference any qualifying conditions* **for application**	• **Types** = *cognitive/conceptual, symbolic &/or instrumental* • **Methods** = *informal or formal; direct or indirect* • **Levels** = *individual, group or department/organization* • **Direct instrumental use:** *change individual behavior (e.g., via assessment tool or Rx intervention options);* **or** *change policy, procedure, protocol, algorithm, program, etc.*	• **Evaluation per type, method, level: e.g., consider conceptual use at individual level**** • **Consider cost-benefit of change + various evaluation efforts** • **Use RU-as-a-process to enhance credibility of evaluation data** • **For both dynamic & pilot evaluations, include:**
• **Affirm/clarify perceived problem/s, with internal and external evidence re: current practice** *[baseline]* • **Consider other influential internal and external factors,** e.g. timelines	• **Critique *systematic reviews and guidelines** • **Re-assess fit of individual sources** • ***Rate the level & quality of each, individual evidence source per a "table of evidence"**	• **Evaluate degree & nature of other criteria:** ****feasibility (r,r,r = risk, resources, readiness);** *pragmatic fit, including potential qualifying factors to application; & nature of **current practice, including the urgency/risk of current issues/needs* • **Make a decision whether/ what to use:** • *Can be a personal practitioner-level decision or a recommendation to others*	• **Cognitive use:** *validate current practice; change personal way of thinking; increase awareness; better understand or appreciate condition/s or experience/s* • **Symbolic use:** *develop position paper or proposal for change; or persuade others regarding a way of thinking* • **CAUTION: Assess whether translation/product or use goes beyond actual findings/evidence:** • *Research evidence may or may not provide various details for a complete policy, procedure, etc.; indicate this fact to users, and note differential levels of evidence therein*	• ***formative, regarding actual implementation & goal progress* • *summative, regarding identified end goal and end-point outcomes*

- **Affirm and focus on high priority issues**
- **Decide if need to form a team, involve formal stakeholders, &/or assign project lead/facilitator**
- **Define desired, measurable outcome/s**
- **Seek out systematic reviews/ guidelines first**
- **Determine need for an explicit type of research evidence, if relevant**
- **Select research sources with** conceptual fit

- **Differentiate statistical and clinical significance**
- **Eliminate non-credible sources**
- **End the process if there is clearly insufficient, credible external evidence that meets your need**

*Stetler, Morsi, Rucki, et al. Appl Nurs Res 1998; 11(4):195–206 for noted tables, reviews, & synthesis process

- *Judge strength of decision; indicate if primarily "research-based"(R-B) or, per hi use of supplemental info, "E-B"; note level of strength of recommendations per related* table; note any qualifying factors that may influence individualized variations*
- **If decision = "Not use" research findings:**
  - *May conduct own research or delay use till additional research done by others*
  - *If still decide to act now, e.g., on evidence of consensus or another basis for practice, consider need for similar planned change and evaluation.*
- **If decision = "Use/ Consider Use," can mean a recommendation for or against a specific practice**

- **Formal dissemination & change strategies should be planned per relevant research and local barriers:**
  - *Passive education is usually not effective as an isolated strategy. Use Dx analysis** & an ***implementation frame- work to develop a plan. Consider multiple strategies: e.g., opinion leaders; interactive education, reminders & audits.*
  - *Focus on context& to enhance sustainability of organizational-related change*
- **Consider need for appropriate, reasoned variation**
- **WITH B, where made a decision to use in the setting:**
  - *With formal use, may need a dynamic evaluation to effectively implement & continuously improve/refine use of best available evidence across units & time*
- **WITH B', where made decision to** consider use & thus obtain **additional, pragmatic info before a final decision:**
  - *With formal consideration, do a pilot project*
  - *With a pilot project, must assess if need IRB review, per relevant institutional criteria*

NOTE: Model applies to all forms of practice, i.e., educational, clinical, managerial, or other; **to use effectively read 2001 & 1994 model papers.**
**Stetler et al, 2006 re: dx analysis
***E.g.: Rogers' re: implications of attributes of a change; Rycroft-Malone et al.&PARIHS (2002) & Green & Krueter's PRECEDE (1992) models re: implementation
&Stetler, 2003 on context
&&Stetler & Caramanica, 2007 on outcomes

- *External evidence*: Primarily, research findings. Also includes both consensus-based national guidelines (i.e., affirmed experience of widely recognized experts) and systematically obtained and published program evaluation/quality data.
- *Internal evidence*: Systematically and locally obtained performance, planning, quality, and outcome data; also, local consensus and individual affirmed experience.

Background and context

The first form of the Stetler model was developed collaboratively by Cheryl Stetler and Gwen Marram (1976), while faculty at the University of Massachusetts, USA. Although it was developed inductively, with no theoretical underpinnings, this original model has since been refined by Stetler three times, primarily while working in hospital settings. Table 3.1 highlights the development and periodic revisions of the model (detailed in cited publications). Revisions were based on both conceptual work and action learning, with the latter involving continuous and, at times systematic, reflection on the part of users.

During the 1970s and early 1980s, engaging nurses in the "use" versus the "conduct" of research at a large teaching hospital was a challenging task. Similar to medical colleagues, the conduct of research was of greater interest to nurses. In spite of this, limited use of the model did occur with some success, and provided insight into the process (Stetler, 1984). Attention was then turned to better understanding the science of knowledge and research utilization (KU/RU) (Stetler, 1985, Stetler & DiMaggio, 1991) and engaging clinical nurse specialists (CNSs) in a developmental, service-based RU Forum (Stetler *et al.*, 1995). It was from these two activities that the 1994 revision of the model emerged. More specifically, CNSs were perceived at the time as the "best-suited practitioners in a service setting to fulfil and to help others fulfil the RU function" (Stetler *et al.*, 1995: 458). The dual purpose of the RU Forum, with CNSs from both a community-based and a large teaching hospital, was to enhance participants' RU knowledge/skills and explore methods of systematically integrating RU into their role (Stetler *et al.*, 1995). The 1976 model was used initially to guide the forum and was systematically and simultaneously reviewed. The "meaning, clarity, and usefulness of each of … (its) judgmental phases were continuously assessed

Table 3.1 Developmental work on the Stetler model and related concepts/processes

Model version by decade	Conceptual/mixed work	Application work
2000s		
• Stetler (2009): Refinement of wording in the two-page EBP model and the table of assumptions. • Stetler (2001b): Update of the model to facilitate evidence-based practice.	• Stetler and Caramanica (2007): Creation of progressive outcomes for evaluation of an evidence-based practice initiative.	• Stetler *et al.* (2003): Prevention of work-related musculoskeletal injuries. • Newell-Stokes *et al.* (2001): Evidence-based procedure for central venous catheters.
1990s		
• Stetler (1994): Refinement of the Stetler/ Marram model for application of research findings to practice.	• Stetler *et al.* (1998a): Defining evidence. • Stetler *et al.* (1998b): Tools and an approach to conducting a utilization-focused integrative review. • Stetler *et al.* (1995): Review of model components by clinical nurse specialists. • Stetler and DiMaggio (1991): A study of research utilization among clinical nurse specialists.	• Stetler *et al.* (1998a): Using the model as a basis for evidence-based practice throughout a service setting. • Stetler *et al.* (1999): A fall prevention program. • Stetler *et al.* (1995): Enhancing research utilization through a forum for clinical nurse specialists.
1980s		
• No revision	• Stetler (1989): A tool for applying the model. • Stetler (1985): Defining the concept of research utilization. • Stetler (1984): Guidelines for an application project.	• Gardner (in Stetler, 1984): Sample application project.

1976: Stetler/Marram model for applicability of research findings in practice.

EBP, evidence-based practice.

in light of a targeted practice issue" (Stetler *et al.*, 1995: 459). The model that emerged (Stetler, 1994a) was "perceived by participants to be more complete and more user friendly than its predecessor" (Stetler *et al.*, 1995: 460). It introduced concepts of alternate types of use, supplemental evidence, underlying assumptions, and contextual and individual influences. Issues regarding synthesis and limiting conditions were also first noted.

The next major phase of development occurred within the context of experiences with the evolution of a broader EBP model, in a teaching hospital (Baystate Medical Center [BMC]) interested in institutionalizing use of evidence into routine practice (Stetler *et al.*, 1998a). The 1994 version served as the conceptual underpinning for this effort and, once again, CNSs were targeted as the core facilitators of RU/EBP. Staff nurses who were interested in EBP and occasionally able to join related activities were deliberately engaged in facilitated and model-related RU/EBP decision making (Stetler *et al.*, 1999).

The experiences and conceptual work that evolved at BMC (Newell-Stokes *et al.*, 2001; Stetler, 1999; Stetler *et al.*, 1998a, b, 1999, 2003) resulted in further model refinements (Stetler, 2001a, b). These included assumptions regarding types of use and contextual/user influences, as well as refinement of various model components relative to the concept of evidence. For example, the concept of appropriate versus inappropriate variation was introduced. Such variation can occur at both the individual and formal group level through "reasoned individualization" (Newell-Stokes *et al.*, 2001; Stetler, 2001b). Further clarification of the synthesis process, related evidence tables, qualifiers of application, and the planned change process occurred. This revision made it clear that the model was applicable "as a critical thinking process, whether used by an individual or by individuals operating within a group" (Stetler, 2001b: 272). This publication was more oriented to organizational use than individual practitioner change; thus readers were referred back to the 1994 model for critical content not repeated, most particularly regarding underlying science and the individual level of use.

Finally, in the late 2000s, two "developments" occurred. An evaluation framework was created, based on the developer's decades of experiences as well as related research and experiences reported in the literature (Stetler and Caramanica, 2007). This framework describes potential outcomes of EBP initiatives at both the individual and group level, per the types of use outlined in the model. Secondly, in preparation for this chapter on the Stetler model, the two-page figure was refined; that is, it was retitled as a model of EBP; significant wording changes were made, particularly to Part II (Fig. 3.1A, B); and the table of assumptions was updated (Table 3.2). These model refinements highlight use of *evidence* and *implementation science concepts*, for example:

(1) *Diagnostic analysis* is an assessment of potential and actual barriers and facilitators, including the context and potential users therein (Stetler, 1994a). Such analysis should occur prior to

Table 3.2 Underlying assumptions of the Stetler model of EBP

Assumptions	Comments/implications
1. Other types of evidence and/or nonresearch-related information are likely to be combined with research findings to facilitate decision making or problem solving.	• Theoretical, experiential, and other forms of information are more likely to be used by individuals and groups to supplement research findings than they are to be ignored. Some of this information may take the form of alternate sources of *evidence*, for example, consensus of national experts (*external* evidence), or local program data and local consensus per affirmed experience (*internal* evidence) (Stetler, 1994, 2001; Stetler *et al.*, 1998a) • It is critical that users understand the strength of various types of evidence (both *individual* sources and as synthesized into a *recommendation*) as well as the difference between "opinion" and affirmed experience (Stetler *et al.*, 1998a).
2. The formal organization may or may not be directly involved in an individual's use of research or other evidence.	• Use by individuals can be directed by the organization through evidence-based policies, procedures, and additional prescriptive documents. • Use of research and other related evidence can also effectively occur informally and routinely at the level of a skilled individual clinician, manager, educator, or other specialist who has relevant competencies and up-to-date knowledge.
3. Utilization may be instrumental, conceptual, and/or symbolic/strategic.	• Use of research findings and other related evidence may be direct and observable or indirect and difficult to identify. Use can change one's way of thinking or influence a direct, observable plan of action. It also can, appropriately or inappropriately, be used to persuade others to shift their thinking and behavior (Stetler, 1994, 2001; Stetler and Caramanica, 2007).

(Continued)

Table 3.2 (*Continued*)

Assumptions	Comments/implications
4. Internal and external factors can influence an individual's or group's view and use of evidence.	• Use of research and related evidence is influenced not only by scientific criteria, but also by (a) the beliefs/attitudes/perceptions, needs, and competencies of individual users and (b) the related context, both local and the environment external to the setting. • Context can either be a barrier or facilitator to use (a) in general (e.g., through culture and availability of resources, such as experts) or (b) specifically (e.g., in terms of an organization's approach to evidence/implementation or contextual factors relevant to a specific innovation) (Stetler, 1994; Stetler *et al.*, 2009).
5. Research, and evaluation, provides us with probabilistic information, not absolutes.	• Findings from research, as well as results from local evaluations, are often expressed in terms of means, standard deviations, or other inferential statistics. Also, at times research provides insights into qualifiers of the application of general findings, such as the potential influence of patient or provider characteristics or settings; and may explain only "some of the variance." Such data do not provide unconditional direction for application to all patients, staff, etc. in all situations. • As a result of qualifiers in research findings and targeted individuals' preferences, needs, experiences, or biological or cultural status, *reasoned variations* from a generally applicable finding may be appropriate; such individualized decision making requires assessment of risk/benefit and related RU/EBP competencies.
6. Lack of knowledge and skills pertaining to research utilization and evidence-based practice in general can inhibit appropriate and effective use.	• Given the complex nature of RU and the often complex nature of practice, the following are essential to effective and safe utilization: knowledge of basic concepts of research and EBP; RU knowledge and skills, including utilization-focused appraisal/synthesis; EBP knowledge and skills, including use of RU/EBP models and tables of evidence; knowledge and interpretive skills regarding inferential statistics and the applicability of findings at the individual level, including appropriate versus inappropriate variation; knowledge of the substantive area under consideration; knowledge of implementation models/frameworks; and critical thinking skills.

Adapted from Stetler (2001b)
EBP, evidence-based practice.

making final plans for implementation (Stetler *et al.*, 2006) and relates to enhancing its success and sustainability.

(2) *Practical implementation concepts and frameworks*, for example, an understanding of the "attributes" of a needed change, such as its complexity (Rogers, 1995); common barriers and facilitators to change, as described in the *Precede-Proceed* framework (Green and Kreuter, 1992); and key factors related to the success of implementation, as in the PARIHS framework (Rycroft-Malone *et al.*, 2002).

The evolutionary changes and pragmatic use of the model in multiple institutions has resulted in not only cited revisions of the model (1994a, 2001b, 2009), but also a related set of published resources (Table 3.3). The Stetler model now, in reality, is a resource toolkit for implementing evidence into practice (see Table 3.3). This is consistent with Haynes' definition of EBP as "a set of tools and resources for finding and applying current best evidence from research …" (Haynes, 2002: 3). As such, it focuses on "a series of judgmental activities about the appropriateness, desirability, feasibility, and manner of … [finding and applying] research findings [and other related evidence] in an individual's or group's practice" (Stetler, 2001b: 272).

Intended audience and actual users of the model

The Stetler/Marram model (1976) was initially created for baccalaureate (BSN) nurses and the general "nurse consumer." However, because of the complexity of the implementation process, Stetler subsequently focused more on advanced practice nurses in autonomous practice with an ability to facilitate other nurses' use of evidence. Actual users of the framework, however, have not been limited to CNSs. The Stetler model consistently has been cited over the years to introduce, update, and engage practicing nurses of all levels in EBP (Morse, 2006; White *et al.*, 2002). In addition, the model has been used by schools of nursing both at the BSN and master's level in and outside of the USA. Radjenovic and Chally (1998), for example, believe that "it is applicable to an individual or organizational process and seem(s) particularly suited for student use." (p. 27). Other users have included the California State University/Northridge (personal communication, 1999, MH); University of Bradford (http://www.brad.ac.uk/acad/health/effprc.htm); and University of Ottawa (http://courseweb.edteched.uottawa.ca/nsg6133/Course_Modules/

Table 3.3 Stetler model: An integrated package of tools/resources for EBP

"How-to" focus	Elements/tools	Source
Utilization-focused reviews	• Individual study evaluation form • Study evaluation tables as part of an overall integrative review: Part I Methodological factors, with instructions; Part II Utilization factors, with instructions • Evaluation forms for existent integrative reviews and meta-analyses	• Stetler *et al.* (1995) for individual focus • Stetler *et al.* (1998b) • Stetler *et al.* (1998b)
Level/strength of evidence	• Strength of reviewed evidence from individual research or other relevant sources (Table) • Strength of an evidence-based recommendation per overall quality and amount of evidence (Table)	• Stetler *et al.* (1998b), Stetler (2001b) – refinement available from author
Synthesis of evidence	• Process steps • Examples	• Stetler *et al.* (1998b), Newell-Stokes *et al.* (2001)

Evaluation regarding use	• Evaluation model for EBP initiatives:
	  • For individual and group levels
	  • Per cognitive, strategic or instrumental use
	• Formative evaluation methods
	  • Diagnostic, implementation-focused, process related and interpretive
	  • Examples
		• Stetler and Caramanica (2007)
		
		• Stetler *et al.* (2006)
		
		• Stetler *et al.* (1999)

Enhancing practitioner level use	• Research utilization forum for engaging and mentoring advanced level nurses	• Stetler *et al.* (1995)
Institutionalization/ organizational support for EBP and model use	• An evolving organizational framework for EBP • Example	• Stetler (2003) • Stetler *et al.* (1998a)
Details regarding use of a specific EBP	• 2009 Visual, Parts I and II • Table of assumptions • Narrative content	• Stetler (2009) • Stetler (2009) • Stetler (1994, 2001)

EBP, evidence-based practice.

Module_PDFs/Stetler-Marram.pdf). In the same vein, the model has appeared in various nursing research, EBP, and related textbooks (e.g., Burns and Grove, 2005; Melynk and Fineout-Overholt, in press; Tiffany and Johnson Lutjens, 1998). Numerous students, both BSN and master's level, continue to write to the developer for permission to use the model and related resources (Table 3.3).

Although the prime target for the model is master's level nurses, it is still viewed as a valuable, although challenging tool, for baccalaureate students. The ability of BSN students to use the model independently is limited given their lack of clinical knowledge and basic knowledge of research methodologies and statistics. Basically, both baccalaureate students and BSNs in practice are capable of understanding the essential premises of the Stetler model. Their education can enable them to understand the skills needed to safely and effectively use research and thus (a) be cautious consumers, especially of individual studies and (b) be cognizant of their own level of need to obtain support or needed skills. Overall, the optimal use of the model with BSN prepared nurses is viewed as the following:

(1) *Use of the model within a facilitated team setting*, facilitated by an advanced practice nurse, affiliated faculty member, or nurse researcher who leads use of the model and oversees and completes final critiques and synthesis of studies (Phase II–III). Staff nurses may participate in various model tasks relative to their ability and available time. For example, staff nurses can and should identify problems or catalysts relative to the potential need for evidence-based change in their practice (Phase I); identify and read relevant papers, as feasible (Phase II); be fully informed by the facilitators regarding synthesized findings, the related process and implications; and provide input into guided applicability discussions, final decision making about use, and implementation planning – building on their clinical expertise and knowledge of both patient experiences/preferences/needs and local context (Phases III and IV); and participate in and facilitate implementation and needed evaluations (Phases IV and V).

(2) *Individual use as appropriate*, but again with support as needed from an advanced practice nurse and/or equivalent clinical expert (e.g., a certified wound care nurse) familiar with the model. Professional nurses should be reflective and engage in clinical inquiry as part of professional practice (Clinical Scholarship Task Force, 1999). As part of that critical role, the model is valuable

given the potential complexity of safe interpretation of individual studies and need for a cautious approach to unsubstantiated recommendations in the literature. For example, professionals should be familiar with competencies and criteria for evaluating applicability of findings and should be cognizant of local context and related expectations, including polices and approaches to reasoned individualization by a staff nurse.

Finally, the Stetler model can be used at the organizational/institutionalization level (Stetler, 2003), as it provides published definitions, values, assumptions, resources, and processes for operationalizing EBP at multiple levels (Stetler *et al.*, 1998a). Although the model could be used at the broader policy level, the author has no direct evidence of such use.

Hypotheses and propositions

To the knowledge of the developer, there has been little comparative or hypothesis-related testing of the model. Formal study of the model as a whole would be complex and challenging, with a need to validate related assumptions. However, individual aspects of the model have been supported in nursing research (Estabrooks, 1999; Stetler and DiMaggio, 1991; Stetler and Caramanica, 2007) and are also supported by current implementation literature (Rycroft-Malone *et al.*, 2004; Stetler *et al.*, 2006; van Achterberg *et al.*, 2008). For example, the literature continues to reinforce the importance of context (McCormack *et al.*, 2002), as well as the potential value of implementation frameworks (Grol *et al.*, 2004). Additionally, the assumption regarding use of other sources of evidence has been echoed by others (CHSRF, 2005).

Use and related evaluation of the Stetler model

The Stetler model has been cited as a "classic model" for RU/EBP (Davies, 2002) and as one of the "most established" (Simpson, 2004). Tiffany and Johnson Lutjens (1998), in a book on planned change, noted that the model was valued by social scientists and nurses. More recently, an introduction to knowledge translation models, strategies, and measures was disseminated to an international audience (Sudsawad, 2007). Sudsawad chose the Stetler model to represent individual-focused frameworks (http://www.ncddr.org/kt/products/ktintro/). Nevertheless, there are few intervention studies that test the Stetler model or indeed other RU/EBP models (Davies, 2002; Mohide and King, 2003). Evidence regarding use of the Stetler model thus comes not from experimental studies but rather from other levels of evidence, as described in the next two sections.

Developer-related evidence

The Stetler model has continuously and systematically been used by master's prepared advanced practice nurses. These experiences provide case reports regarding the model's application at multiple levels in multiple settings, from the 1980s onward. There are also publications describing projects with a formal evaluation component. Specifically, developer-related uses of the Stetler model have been reported as follows:

- Case report by a neuro nurse specialist: Describes development and dissemination of a "set of guidelines which establishes timed interventions for nutritional support of the severely head-injured patients in the neuro intensive care unit" at Massachusetts General Hospital (MGH) (Stetler, 1984: 5–87).
- Case report by a nurse manager: Recorded in a reflective evaluation interview videotaped at MGH, focused on tube feedings, diarrhea, and research-based practice guidelines for staff; results were mixed (Stetler, 1984: 5–11).
- Case report by a CNS (Stetler, 1994b): Use of a single study regarding an assessment tool for out-patient care, after a period of "considered use," to educate a young pregnant woman to successfully monitor lack of fetal movement.
- Case reports by three CNSs, based at two different hospitals, with multiple examples of positive change and influence on decisions and actions (Stetler *et al.*, 1995): Overall evaluation by 13 CNSs of the related RU Forum indicated objectives to enhance knowledge and skill were moderately positive, with scores significantly influenced by the "level of participation." One factor influencing the scores, as one CNS said, was that she "knows less now that she knows more." (Stetler *et al.*, 1995: 463). Another CNS, however, articulated the overall essence of the change as:

    a better overall picture of the applicability of findings for practice. Before this education in RU, it took me forever to review an article, never mind what I would do with the results! ... With this new approach, I find research 'friendlier' to consider for its use in my day-to-day practice, and I am better able to influence and support staff nurses in making clinical decisions (p. 466).

- Case reports by two additional CNSs, at BMC, as described through exemplars of clinical scholarship (Stetler, 1999): Aspects of the model and related resources are referenced in the exemplars, for example, "One step that I took in this decision making process was to evaluate the CAGE based on criteria for assessing the applicability of research findings for practice."
- Formative and summative evaluation of a falls prevention program: Formative data involved observation via rounding, staff surveys, audit/feedback, and a focus group. Key stakeholders viewed the evidence-based falls program as useful; and outcomes evaluation indicated:

the absolute [falls] rate was at the lower, positive end in comparison to rates reported by other institutions in the literature. More importantly, we saw a clear decline in the level of severity of patient-related fall injuries (Stetler *et al.*, 1999).

- Evaluation of a central line project (Newell-Stokes *et al.*, 2001): Involved a process audit that indicated overall "good" compliance with a policy/procedure change, although related data collection was less than optimal. It also included on-going, informal monitoring regarding infection-related problems, including communication with the Infection Control office. Peripherally inserted central catheter (PICC) data indicated some noncompliance in the ICU relative to a preferred use of heparin, as well as difficulties in home care. Thanks to careful monitoring in the latter, a problem was quickly identified and steps taken. In hindsight, the model was not an issue but rather input from key stakeholders should have been pursued more aggressively to assess "fit" in home care. Inpatient results were considered successful and, overall, the importance of model components was actually reinforced.
- Report of an evidence-based management program to prevent musculoskeletal injuries (Stetler *et al.*, 2003): At the time of publication, after departure of the developer, the work was still in progress. Reports from those still at BMC suggested that goal-oriented accomplishments were notable; for example, there was mandatory flexibility and stretching exercises for patient handlers and a downward trend in injury rates.

After 2000, the developer was no longer in the service setting. Her direct access to and influence on the collection of evaluative evidence of the model's use and effectiveness was thus severely curtailed.

Evidence from others

A review of the literature and the web illustrate a number of "uses" of the model, as does a more limited set of personal communications with the developer. "Evaluation" is an elusive aspect of many of these uses, with the *choice* of the model in some cases being the only indicator of "success" or perceived "usefulness."

To begin, there are a number of publications that describe how the Stetler model has been used over the years on an international basis. However, a number of them do not seem to actually implement targeted findings/interventions. For example, a number of authors have used the model as a framework to guide review of the literature and to "develop" an intervention or, at minimum, implications for practice (Bradish *et al.*, 1996; Bauer *et al.*, 2002; Cole *et al.*, 2006). Specific examples include Christie and Moore (2005), using the 2001 version, who felt their "in-depth" review had "implications for nurses because humour can be an effective intervention"; and Lefler (2002), using the 1994 version, who developed specific implications for practice in terms of both cognitive (e.g., raise awareness) and instrumental use for advanced practice nurses.

A number of accessible reports regarding the model's broader use in both academic and clinical settings are listed in Table 3.4. The clinical settings included acute care, ambulatory, and long-term care. "Users" were faculty, advanced practice nurses, and staff. Some authors concurred with the developer that clinical nursing staff could use the model with assistance from an educator, CNS, or nurse researcher. One project tested the model (Uitterhoeve and Ambaum, 1999) using a unique, qualitative approach; that is, using Donabedian's structure, process and outcome framework. They established criteria for each phase and then assessed achievement of those criteria. Their conclusion was that the model "... proved to be a very useful vehicle through which to promote the use of research findings." Furthermore, the Stetler model "... not only facilitated the application of research findings, but also educated practicing nurses in research methodology and critique" (Uitterhoeve and Ambaum, 1999: 191).

Table 3.4 Additional uses of the Stetler model reported in the published literature

Source[a]	Focus/results	Comments

1. McGuire (1992): The process of implementing research into clinical practice. Proceedings of the Second National Oncology Nursing Forum, Conference on Cancer Nursing Research.
a. RU program at the Johns Hopkins Oncology Center Department of Nursing used the Stetler/Marram model and then the 1994 update as their framework.
b. Two overview papers: McGuire *et al.* (1994a, b).
	• Reedy *et al.* (1994): Project on amphotericin B – facilitated development of protocol and standing orders that were implemented.
	• Hanson and Ashley (1994): Project on bereavement care–resulted in organizational and clinical recommendations to improve bereavement care.
	• Shelton *et al.*, 1997: Recommendation made to staff, reportedly with some positive effects (abstract only)
		• Two published projects and an abstract from a student project reflect the model's use at this comprehensive cancer center.
		• Projects lead primarily by CNSs.
		• Perceptions of use:
		  • "Staff nurses can use the Stetler-Marram model but need resources and support from individuals, committees, and administration" (Reedy *et al.*, 1994: 715).
		  • "The Stetler model facilitates implementation of research findings into clinical nursing practice" (Hanson and Ashley, 1994: 720).

2. Specht *et al.* (1995): Adoption of a research-based practice for treatment of pressure ulcers.	• Evaluation of a skin care protocol per chart audits showed "notable changes." • Practitioners adopted the research-based practice; accompanied by decreased costs.	• Large long-term care facility with primary nursing. • Strong staff nurse participation in the RU change. • 1994 version • Balanced individualized decision making with research-based parameters for the decisions • Consulted with a nurse expert.

Table 3.4 *(Continued)*

Source[a]	Focus/results	Comments
3. Gaskamp (1997): Teaching research utilization in a baccalaureate nursing program.	• "… better results in students, with a greater understanding of and enthusiasm toward research and higher regard for participating in research utilization" (p. 39)	• 1976 version as the framework for the course.
4. Radjenovic and Chally (1998): Research utilization and undergraduate students.	• Integrated an active, instrumental RU focus into a senior level clinical BSN course.	• 1994 version and the basic utilization-focused critique tool (Stetler, 1989). • Users recognized the model's advanced level focus but felt relevant for students with faculty and nursing staff's expertise.
5. Uitterhoeve and Ambaum (1999): Surviving the era of evidence-based nursing practice: Implementation of a research utilization model in practice.	• Tested model using Donabedian's structure, process, and outcome framework. • Goal of the process: achieve a knowledge update for staff concerning incidence and prevalence of psychosocial issues in specific patients. • Goal was "perceived to have been met" (p. 191)	• 1994 version. • Out-patient clinic of a University Hospital in the Netherlands. • Included staff nurses; group facilitated/lead by CNS • Focus was conceptual use
6. White *et al.* (2002): Using evidence to educate birthing center nursing staff regarding infant states, cues, and behaviors.	• Focused on application of targeted evidence after a review of the literature. • "Post-test results indicated that the staff's knowledge and skill related to interpreting infant behavior to parents increased" (p. 298) [Average change = 1.47 points on six-point scale].	• 1994 model. • Focus = Birthing center nursing staff and prenatal parenting instructors. • Women's health center.

(Continued)

Table 3.4 (*Continued*)

Source[a]	Focus/results	Comments
7. Tsai (2003): The effects of a research utilization in-service program on nurses.	• Eight-week extensive RU in-service course. • Stetler model as framework. • Slightly more positive results for attitude but no RU change. • Lack of feasibility and the needed research for identified problems = potential issues; also contextual problems.	• Taiwan medical center. • 1994 version. • Nurses had at least 1 year of experience; mixed education backgrounds (63% university-based) • "… results suggest that continuous consultation and assistance should be provided after the course" (Tsai, p. 105)

EBP, evidence-based practice; RU, research utilization; CNS, clinical nurse specialist, BNS, baccalaureate.

[a]Unless otherwise specified, articles in the table are USA based.

Other papers (Table 3.4) provided various types of evidence regarding the success of related projects or perceptions of the model's value. Project reports were generally positive, but did not always focus on actual behavior. Tsai (2003) used an RU survey, said to have validity, but did not find an effect from extensive education. She noted a number of potential barriers, including the need to provide consultative support as follow-up to clinically based education. Overall, the type of use described in these projects was cognitive (e.g., knowledge or attitude) and instrumental. Of interest is the approach of Specht *et al.* (1995), who used balanced individualized decision making with formal, research-based parameters for related decisions.

In addition to the examples of use in the preceding text, other evidence is available that the Stetler model has been used as the framework for various academic theses and clinical projects. At times, follow-up implementation is noted but not explicitly reported. Knowledge of such use comes through communications with the developer, presentations at conferences, or web postings; for example, Blahovich (2006) reported use of the 2001 model to guide a VAP-related project; and, through personal communication, a student (NS) described use of the model in 2007 for a professional project/paper:

> *The model's step by step process secured my ideas (so jumbled in the beginning) in the right path to make sense. However, the proposed 'order set' for febrile neutropenia is kind of on hold for now because of various reasons at my workplace.*

Access to such "gray literature," even in abstract form, is extremely difficult and limited. Follow-up requests are rarely successful.

Other sample uses are as follows:

- The model was cited as the focus of a hospital-based program first developed in 2004 (http://www.nyp.org/nursing/resources); for example,

> *This has been a learning opportunity as well as a significant step in the pursuit of continued excellence and the promotion of evidence based practice in nursing. Members have been developing expertise in the review of nursing research proposals and the use of the Stetler Model in the research utilization process.*

- Based on the 1994 model and other related citations, as well as "expressed needs of nurses and health care agencies in British Columbia, a decision-making model for utilization of research findings in practice was developed and published in [a] workbook". (Clarke, 1995; also see http://classweb.gmu.edu/rfeeg/ichna/clarke.html)
- In a professional newsletter, the model was cited as providing "a framework to enhance the use of research and evidence to create formal change in practice and critical thinking (Stetler, 2001b). Many areas of patient care have been improved by this method ..." (Sharpe, 2006).
- A collaborative project "... explored the applicability of using the Stetler Model of Research Utilization strategy in China" (Decker *et al.*, 2007). It was based on collaboration between Saginaw Valley State University in the USA, and Jinan University Hospital in China "to further the knowledge of evidence based practice (EBP) in professional nurses and students in both agencies."

In summary, the model and its related tools have reportedly been used, internationally, to enhance cognitive and instrumental outcomes. However, rigorous testing has yet to occur. Support for its usefulness is thus conceptual, per its grounding in KU/implementation science; and, additionally, is enhanced by the following sources:

- Its affirmation by various CNSs with whom the author directly worked in four institutions.
- Other developer-related publications describing use of the model with useful outcomes.
- Periodic reports of its use by others, per publications or web site postings.
- Continued requests to the author for various academic, clinical, and professional uses of the model or related resources.

Perceived strengths and weaknesses of the model

Strengths

The developer identifies major strengths of the Stetler model as its practitioner orientation, critical thinking focus, grounding in KU and implementation science, and its strong relationship to the experiences of advanced level practitioners in the real world of application. Although other models may focus on critical thinking, at least implicitly, the Stetler model's goal is to make the process of decision making regarding use of evidence explicit and transparent for the user, be that an individual practitioner or a group of practitioners making a collective decision. This includes critical thinking throughout various phases of the RU/EBP process, in terms of the following:

- Nature of the problem and desired outcomes.
- Nature of acceptable evidence.
- Acceptable level of overall strength of acceptable evidence.
- Applicability of acceptable evidence.
- Nature of the evidence-based change or innovation, including type of use.
- Nature of the influence of context and potential users on application, relative to barriers and facilitators.
- Nature of implementation and evaluation, relative to type of use and outcomes desired.

Another perceived strength is the explicit direction provided for users through an integrated package of tools/resources, including related examples, designed to facilitate decision making/critical thinking (Table 3.3). The model thus provides assistance in, for example, doing utilization-focused critiques, synthesizing evidence, and identifying alternate outcomes across different levels of users. Other strengths are the model's explicit recognition of alternate types/ sources of evidence; alternate uses of evidence (i.e., not only concrete use); and its grounding in an explicit set of assumptions. Again from the developer's point of view, the model can easily be used as a supplement by advanced level nurses for use with other EBP models that may be perceived as more "user-friendly" by staff.

In terms of others' views, Kennedy and Carr (2005) thought it made "EBP more focused and acceptable to those clinicians who assert, 'This is the way we have always done it.'" At Johns Hopkins, with use of the model, advanced level nurses felt "more comfortable and confident in assuming their research utilization role at both the individual and organizational level" (Hanson and Ashley., 1994: 721), while McClinton (1997) felt that it was a practical model. Nolan *et al.* (1994) noted that the model addresses "characteristics of the clinician who may use research findings" (p. 206); and, like Bradish *et al.* (1996), they recognized that its use is not limited to clinicians. Finally, it has been cited by a predominantly medical research group as one of two conceptual models found "... helpful in providing clear explanations for specific aspects of implementation research that promote external validity, and also bear on human subjects protection issues" (Chaney *et al.*, 2008: 9).

Finally, the Stetler model can be assumed to have perceived validity to others, as it has been repeatedly included in relevant texts for over 30 years. Most recently, Melynk and Fineout-Overholt included it in their first and second edition EBP book (2005; in press). As part of a nonnursing publication, the model was selected to help supplement the Canadian Institute of Health Research (CIHR) knowledge translation model (Sudsawad, 2007). It was the only supplement selected to represent "individual-focused models" and seemingly is one of the few so focused in nursing.

Weaknesses

Limitations relate to its lack of rigorous testing, which of course does not distinguish it from other models, and its complexity. However, given the complexity of KU and implementation, it seems better to recognize challenges up front and deal with them accordingly. On occasion, others have determined that other models are preferable; for example, after comparing it with 22 other models, the Stetler model was not selected as the model of choice by a committee at a large tertiary hospital system focused on promoting "EBP among direct care nurses" (Mohide and King, 2003). The model was ranked among the top eight, based on selected criteria deemed relevant to clinical nursing in their setting, but was not rated sufficiently high on the following criteria: clear and concise, comprehensive, or ease of use by clinicians.

Additionally, some users of the 1976 version felt there was insufficient focus on a specific problem or related questioning (Bradish *et al.*, 1996; Grinspun *et al.*, 1993). Grinspun *et al.* (1993) added a preliminary "questioning" phase to encourage better consideration of the problem. Ultimately, the 1994/2001/2009 versions of the Stetler model include an expanded "preparation" phase.

The fact that the model has several versions has meant that users do not always utilize the most recent version (see Table 3.4) or do not recognize the full potential or scope of the model. The model is designed primarily for a skilled individual for whom such use should be routine; and without targeted critical thinking at that level, application of research may become a task oriented, mechanistic routine that can lead to inappropriate, ineffective, or nonevidence-based practice at the individual patient level. Finally, there are those who recognize that the model, in whatever version, can be difficult for staff nurses; for example, Reedy *et al.* (1994) noted that the "Stetler-Marram model helped staff nurses decide how to apply research findings to practice, although using it was difficult and required mentorship." This is not unexpected, as the same authors later note that "staff nurses can use the Stetler-Marram model but need resources and support from individuals, committees, and administration," an observation with which the developer agrees, particularly as it has evolved in complexity.

Information on barriers and facilitators to implementing the model

Barriers and facilitators are basically defined by reviewing the above limitations and strengths, as well as the model's assumptions (Table 3.2). Barriers are created by the complexity of the model and its multiple versions. Without the willingness to explore in-depth the integrated package of the Stetler model and its details, its use will not be optimized (Table 3.3); for example, consider those settings that use information on identifying the strength of *individual sources* of evidence but do not follow through in their decision making/critical thinking regarding implications of the strength of the *final recommendation/s* that emerge from a synthesis of the overall, and usually mixed levels, of evidence. Barriers are also created if those in a position to role model or mentor others have not had hands-on, reflective experience with the model. Finally, it is a barrier to expect staff nurses to use the model without sufficient expert support. Experiences in various hospitals suggest that staff can successfully participate and use a framework, such as the Stetler model, but benefit from (a) preparatory critique and synthesis work by experts, such as nurse researchers or CNSs; (b) networking with professional associations, and (c) on-going support and consultation. Staff can thus engage in focused, meaningful decision making about RU/EBP (Stetler and Caramanica, 2007; Stetler *et al.*, 1998b); and those who are interested can delve more deeply into the model and related details. Again, if a simpler looking model is needed for staff, this does not obviate use of the Stetler model to supplement, facilitate and support critical decision making and RU/EBP operationalization.

In terms of facilitators, in addition to consultation and mentoring from advanced level nurses or other experts (Stetler *et al.*, 1995), and the integrated package of tools/resources, facilitators to use of the Stetler model include the following:

- Appropriate education at the undergraduate and graduate levels (Radjenovic and Chally, 1998), as well as clinically based educational programs with interactive follow-up (Tsai, 2003).
- A supportive context that provides mentors or consultants (Reedy *et al.*, 1994; Tsai, 2003), as well as other organizational resources such as staff time for mentoring/development and related project work (Stetler, 2003; Stetler *et al.*, 1998a).

In summary, for a service setting wishing to support critical thinking and professional practice, the Stetler model, with related resources and a supportive, reflective context, can enhance the ability to "better implement conscious, deliberate, research-based nursing practice" (Stetler *et al.*, 1995: 46).

The future

At this point in time, the developer does not have any plans for testing the model. However, she would urge others, from those involved in doctoral work to those who use it in clinical settings, to engage in formative and summative evaluations that provide insights regarding an array of questions and issues; for example:

- To what extent do assumptions need to be met for ease of use and successful outcomes?
- Which, if any, components of the model influence the nature of day-to-day decision making and consultation of CNSs or others at the master's level well familiar with the model?
- To what extent does the model provide answers/directions to questions and issues that arise in efforts to implement evidence into practice?

In the end, the Stetler model is a sequential but interactive series of critical thinking and criteria-based decision-making steps. Ultimately, the model's steps or phases are designed to facilitate effective use of research and other best available evidence. It is hoped that there are nursing scholars interested in assessing (a) the degree to which the model's components influence achievement of that goal and (b) the related factors that influence achievement in terms of specific types of use, specific types of users, the circumstances of use, and the related nature of the context.

Summary

- Primarily, for use by *advanced level practitioners* (nurse or other), in terms of their own use of evidence and facilitation of use by others – at the individual and group level; this requires exploration of the 1994 version, focused primarily on use by an EBP competent individual, *and* the 2009 version, focused more broadly on use by a group/team of individuals (uni- or inter-disciplinary).
- For use by BSN prepared nurses primarily *within a facilitated team setting*; also for *individual BSN use as appropriate*, that is, with needed support from an advanced level nurse and/or equivalent clinical expert familiar with the model.
- For use by a *department/organization*, as a guiding EBP framework in terms of its published definitions, values, assumptions, resources, and processes for operationalizing EBP at multiple levels.

- For use of evidence by knowledgeable *clinicians, academic* and *clinical educators, managers,* and various *specialists,* in terms of improving their own and others' practice; and by *researchers,* for exploration of EBP and implementation.
- For use by *evaluators,* in terms of identifying alternate types of use (cognitive/conceptual, instrumental, and strategic/symbolic) and related outcomes, across different types and levels of users.

References

Bauer, N., Bushey, F., and Maros, D. (2002). Diffusion of responsibility and pressure ulcers. *World Council of Enterostomal Therapists Journal,* 22, 9–17.

Birch, J. (1979). Nursing should be a research-based profession. *Nursing Times,* 2775 (Suppl. 33), 135–136.

Blahovich, M. (2006). *Prevention of Ventilator-Associated Pneumonia by Oral Care Hygiene.* Sigma Theta Tau International Conference 2006. (http://www.nursinglibrary.org/Portal/main.aspx?pageid = 4024&pid = 15442)

Bloch, D. (1979). Nursing research centers. *Nursing Research,* 28, 138.

Bradish, G., Goddard, P., Hatcher, S., *et al.* (1996). Applying the Stetler-Marram model to a nursing administration problem: A graduate student learning experience. *Canadian Journal of Nursing Administration,* 9, 57–70.

Burns, N. and Grove, S. (2005). *The practice of nursing research: Conduct, critique and utilization.* Elsevier Saunders, Philadelphia, PA.

Chaney, E., Rabuck, L.G., Uman, J., *et al.* (2008). Human subjects protection issues in QUERI implementation research: QUERI Series. *Implementation Science,* 5, 10.

Christie, W. and Moore, C. (2005). The impact of humor on patients with cancer. *Clinical Journal of Oncology Nursing,* 9, 211–218.

CHSRF – Lomas, J., Culyer, T., McCutcheon, C., McAuley, L., and Law, S. . (2005). *Conceptualizing and Combining Evidence for Health System Guidance.* Canadian Health Services Research Foundation (http://www.chsrf.ca/).

Ciliska, D., DiCenso, A., Melnyk, B., and Stetler, C. (2005). Using models and strategies for evidence-based practice. In: *Evidence-based Practice in Nursing and Healthcare: A guide for Translating Research Evidence into Best Practice* (eds, B. Melynk and E. Fineout-Overholt), 1st edn, pp. 185–219. Lippincott Williams & Wilkins, Philadelphia, PA.

Clinical Scholarship Task Force. (1999). *Clinical scholarship white paper: Knowledge work, in service of care, based on evidence.* Sigma Theta Tau International, Indianapolis, IN.

Cole, K., Waldrop, J., D'Auria, J., Garner, H. (2006). An integrative research review: Effective school-based childhood overweight interventions. *Journal of Specialty Pediatric Nursing,* 11, 166–177.

Davies, B.L. (2002). Sources and models for moving research evidence into clinical practice. *Journal of Obstetrical Gynecological Neonatal Nursing*, 31(5), 558–562.

Decker, S.A., Shannon, M., Roe, E., Lin, Q., and Wieju, C. (2007). *Global Collaboration for Culturally Competent Care: Strategies to Support EBP*. International Nursing Research Congress Focusing on Evidence-Based Practice (http://www.svsu.edu/2008-edition/nursing/sally-a-decker.html).

Diers, D. (1972). Application of research to nursing practice. *Image*, 5, 7–11.

Estabrooks, C.A. (1999). The conceptual structure of research utilization. *Research in Nursing and Health*, 22, 203–216.

Gaskamp, C.D. (1997). Teaching research utilization in a baccalaureate nursing program. *Nurse Educator*, 22, 39.

Graham, I. and Tetroe, J. (2009). Planned action theories. In: *Knowledge Translation in Health Care* (eds, S. Straus, K. Tetroe, and I. Graham), pp. 185–195. Wiley Blackwell & BMJ Books, Oxford.

Green, L.W. and Kreuter, M.W. (1992). CDC's planned approach to community health as an application of PRECEDE and an inspiration for PROCEED. *Journal of Health Education*, 23, 140–147.

Grinspun, D., MacMillan, K., Nichol, H., and Shields-Poë, D. (1993). Using research findings in the hospital. *Canadian Nurse*, 89, 46–48.

Grol, R., Wensing, M., and Eccles, M. (2004). *Improving Patient Care: The Implementation of Change in Clinical Practice* (Elsevier Health Sciences). Elsevier, Oxford, UK.

Gunter, L.M. (1971). [Encouraging utilization of research findings in nursing]. *Kango Kenkyu*, 4, 315–321 [article in Japanese].

Hanson, J.L. and Ashley, B. (1994). Advanced practice nurses' application of the Stetler model for research utilization: Improving bereavement care. *Oncology Nursing Forum*, 21, 720–724.

Harrison, S.P. (1978). [Nursing research: Nursing a research-directed profession]. *Sygeplejersken*, 78, 4–6 [article in Danish].

Haynes, R.B. (2002). What kind of evidence is it that evidence-based medicine advocates want health care providers and consumers to pay attention to? *BMC Health Services Research*, 2, 3f.

Kennedy, H.P. and Carr, K.C. (2005). Conceptual adaptation of the Stetler Model. In: *Women's Gynecologic Health* (eds, K. Schuiling and F. Likis). Jones & Bartlett, Boston, MA.

Kim, S. (1999). Models of theory-practice linkage in nursing. Presented at International Nursing Research Conference: Research to Practice. University of Alberta, Edmonton, Canada.

Lefler, L. (2002). The advanced practice nurse's role regarding women's delay in seeking treatment with myocardial infarction. *Journal of American Academy of Nurse Practitioners*, 14, 449–456.

McClinton, J. (1997). Stetler model of research utilization. Masters in Public Administration (http://www.kumc.edu/instruction/nursing/NRSG754/SYLLABUS/stetlermodel.html).

McCormack, B., Kitson, A., Harvey. G., Rycroft-Malone, J., Titchen, A., and Seers K. (2002). Getting evidence into practice: The meaning of 'context'. *Journal of Advanced Nursing*, 38(1), 94–104.

McGuire, D., Walczak, J.R., Krumm, W.L., *et al.* (1994a). Research utilization in oncology nursing: Application of the Stetler Model in a comprehensive cancer center. *Oncology Nursing Forum*, 21, 703–704.

McGuire, D., Walczak, J.R., and Krumm, W.L. (1994b). Development of a nursing research utilization program in a clinical oncology setting: Organization, implementation, and evaluation. *Oncology Nursing Forum*, 21, 704–710.

McGuire, D. (1992). The process of implementing research into clinical practice. *Proceedings of the Second National Oncology Nursing Forum, Conference on Cancer Nursing Research*. American Cancer Society: Atlanta.

Melynk, B. and Fineout-Overholt, E. (Eds). (2005). *Evidence-based Practice in Nursing and Healthcare: A Guide for Translating Research Evidence into Best Practice* 1st edn. Lippincott Williams & Wilkins, Philadelphia, PA.

Melynk, B. and Fineout-Overholt, E. (Eds). (In press). *Evidence-based Practice in Nursing and Healthcare: A Guide for Best Practice*, 2nd edn. Lippincott Williams & Wilkins, Philadelphia, PA.

Mohide, E.A. and King, B. (2003). Building a foundation for evidence-based practice: Experiences in a tertiary hospital. *Evidence-Based Nursing*, 6, 100–103.

Morse, K. (2006). Editorial: Evidence-based practice links research, experience, patient needs. *Nursing 2008 Critical Care*, 1, 6–6.

Newell-Stokes, V., Broughton, S., Giuliano, K.K., and Stetler, C. (2001). Developing an evidence-based procedure: Maintenance of central venous catheters. *Clinical Nurse Specialist*, 15, 199–206.

Nolan, M.T., Larson, E., McGuire, D., Hill, M.N., and Haller, K. (1994). A review of approaches to integrating research and practice. *Applied Nursing Research*, 7, 199–207.

Radjenovic, D. and Chally, P.S. (1998). Research utilization by undergraduate students. *Nurse Educator*, 23, 26–29.

Reedy, A.M., Shivnan, J.C., Hanson, J.L., Haisfield, M.E., and Gregory, R.E. (1994). The clinical application of research utilization: Amphotericin B. *Oncology Nursing Forum*, 21, 715–719.

Rogers, E.M. (1995). *Diffusion of Innovations*, 4th edn. Free Press, New York.

Rycroft-Malone, J. and Stetler, C. (2004). Commentary on evidence, research, knowledge: A call for conceptual clarity, S. Scott-Findlay, C. Pollock. *Worldviews in Evidence-based Nursing*, 1, 98f.

Rycroft-Malone, J., Kitson, A., Harvey, G., *et al.* (2002). Ingredients for change: Revisiting a conceptual framework. *Quality in Safety and Health Care*, 11, 174–180.

Rycroft-Malone, J., Harvey, G., Seers, K., *et al.* (2004). An exploration of the factors that influence the implementation of evidence into practice. *Journal of Clinical Nursing*, 13, 913–924.

Sharpe, D. (2006). IV extravasations. *Carolina Breaths: North Carolina Association of PeriAnesthesia Nurses*, 23, 5f.

Shelton, B., Bare, J. and Birtwistle, S.J. (1997). Applying the Stetler research utilization (RU) model to evaluate the practice of normal saline instillation (NSI) in cancer patients [abstract]. *American Journal of Critical Care*, 6, 251.

Simpson, R. (2004). Evidence-based nursing offers certainty in the uncertain world of healthcare. *Nursing Management*, 35, 10–12.

Specht, J.P., Bergquist, S. and Frantz, R.A. (1995). Adoption of a research-based practice for treatment of pressure ulcers. *Nursing Clinics of North America*, 30, 553–563.

Stetler, C. (1984). *Nursing Research in a Service Setting*. Reston Publishing Co., Inc., Virginia.

Stetler, C. (1985). Research utilization: Defining the concept. *Image*, 17, 40–44.

Stetler, C. (1989). A strategy for teaching research utilization. *Nurse Educator*, 13, 17–20.

Stetler, C. (1994a). Refinement of the Stetler/Marram model for application of research findings to practice. *Nursing Outlook*, 42, 15–25.

Stetler, C. (1994b). Using research to improve patient care. In: *Nursing Research: Methods, Critical Appraisal, and Utilization* (eds, G. LoBiondo-Wood and J. Haber), 2nd edn. Mosby, St. Louis, MO.

Stetler, C. (1999). Clinical scholarship exemplars: The Baystate Medical Center. In: Clinical Scholarship Task Force's *Clinical Scholarship White Paper: Knowledge Work, in Service of Care, based on Evidence*. Sigma Theta Tau International, Indianapolis, IN.

Stetler, C. (2001a). *Evidence-based Practice and the Use of Research: A Synopsis of Basic Concepts & Strategies to Improve Care*. NOVA Foundation, Washington, D.C. (Out of print)

Stetler, C. (2001b). Updating the Stetler model of research utilization to facilitate evidence-based practice. *Nursing Outlook*, 49, 272–278.

Stetler, C. (2003). The role of the organization in translating research into evidence-based practice. *Outcomes Management for Nursing Practice*, 7, 97–103.

Stetler, C. and Caramanica, L. (2007). Evaluation of an evidence-based practice initiative: Outcomes, strengths and limitations of a retrospective, conceptually-based approach. *Worldviews on Evidence-Based Nursing*, 4, 187–199.

Stetler, C. and DiMaggio, G. (1991). Research utilization among clinical nurse specialists. *Clinical Nurse Specialist*, 5, 151–155.

Stetler, C. and Marram, G. (1976). Evaluating research findings for applicability in practice. *Nursing Outlook*, 24, 559–563.

Stetler, C., Bautista, C., Vernale-Hannon, C., and Foster, J. (1995). Enhancing research utilization by clinical nurse specialists. *Nursing Clinics of North America*, 30, 457–473.

Stetler, C., Brunell, M., Giuliano, K., *et al.* (1998a). Evidence-based practice and the role of nursing leadership. *Journal of Nursing Administration*, 28, 45–53.

Stetler, C., Morsi, D., Rucki, S., *et al.* (1998b). Utilization-focused integrative reviews in a nursing service. *Applied Nursing Research*, 11, 195–206.

Stetler, C., Corrigan, B., Sander-Buscemi, K., and Burns, M. (1999). Integration of evidence into practice and the change process: A fall prevention program as a model. *Outcomes Management for Nursing Practice*, 3/3, 102–111.

Stetler, C., Burns, M., Sander-Buscemi, K., Morsi, D., and Grunwald, E. (2003). Use of evidence for prevention of work-related musculo-skeletal injuries. *Orthopaedic Nursing*, 22, 32–41.

Stetler, C., Legro, M., Wallace, C., *et al.* (2006). The role of formative evaluation in implementation research and the QUERI experience. *Journal of General Internal Medicine*, 21 (Suppl. 2), S1–S8.

Stetler, C., Ritchie, J.A., Rycroft-Malone, J., Schultz, A.A., and Charns, M.P. (2009). Institutionalizing evidence-based practice: An organizational case study using a model of strategic change. *Implementation Science*, 4, 78.

Stetler, C. (2010). Stetler model. In: *Models and frameworks for implementing evidence-based practice* (eds, J. Rycroft-Malone and T. Bucknall), pp. 51–80. Wiley-Blackwell, Oxford, UK.

Sudsawad, P. (2007). *Knowledge translation: Introduction to models, strategies, and measures.* Southwest Educational Development Laboratory, National Center for the Dissemination of Disability Research, Austin, TX.

Tiffany, C.T. and Johnson Lutjens, L.R. (1998). *Planned Change Theories for Nursing: Review, Analysis, and Implications.* Sage Publications, Thousand Oaks, CA.

Tsai, S.-L. (2003). The effects of a research utilization in-service program on nurses. *International Journal of Nursing Studies*, 40, 105–113.

Uitterhoeve, R. and Ambaum, B. (1999). Surviving the era of evidence-based nursing practice: Implementation of a research utilization model in practice. *European Journal of Oncology Nursing*, 3, 185–191.

van Achterberg, T., Schoonhoven, L., and Grol, R. (2008). Nursing implementation science: How evidence-based nursing requires evidence-based implementation. *Journal of Nursing Scholarship*, 40, 302–310.

White, C., Simon, M., and Bryan, A. (2002). Using evidence to educate birthing center nursing staff: About infant states, cues, and behaviors. *MCN, American Journal of Maternal Child Nursing*, 27, 294–298.

Chapter 4

The Ottawa Model of Research Use

Jo Logan and Ian D. Graham

Key learning points

- The Ottawa Model of Research Use (OMRU) offers a comprehensive, interdisciplinary framework of elements that affect the process of getting valid research findings applied in practice.
- The OMRU is a planned action model and its purpose is to assist facilitators to implement valid research into practice. It is both descriptive and prescriptive.
- The model is comprised of six elements that are central to the process of research use: the research-informed innovation, the potential adopters, the practice environment, implementation interventions for transferring the research findings into practice, the adoption of the innovation, and the health-related and other outcomes.
- The prescriptive aspect of the model is the assessment, monitoring, and evaluation (AME) process.
- The OMRU may be applied at any level in the delivery of care (e.g., individual or team), organizational (unit, department, hospital), or health care system. The AME portion of the OMRU is of particular use to those in practice settings, while the structural portion of the model's six elements can provide a basis to scientists in their work.

This chapter presents our latest thinking about the Ottawa Model of Research Use (OMRU) (Graham and Logan, 2004a, 2006; Logan and Graham, 1998). There has been significant growth in the research use field since we first published it in 1998, subsequently the OMRU has been used both in research and practice. As a result, we have updated the model and will share some reflections and pose possible future directions.

Purpose and assumptions

The OMRU offers a comprehensive, interdisciplinary framework of elements that affect the process of getting valid research findings applied in practice. The purpose of the OMRU is to assist facilitators to implement valid research into practice. It is both descriptive and prescriptive. It presents a pragmatic approach that outlines both the key elements involved and a useful process to guide implementation. OMRU can be classified as a planned action model.

We consider research use to be an interactive synergistic process of interconnected decisions and actions by different individuals related to each of the model elements (Logan and Graham, 1998). The model is dynamic, meaning that we assume that each element influences and is influenced by the others. This is depicted by double arrows that create multiple feedback loops (Fig. 4.1). The process takes place over time and in an order that depends on the status of each element within the specific context. The model has been influenced by a social constructivist perspective originating from our nursing educational and sociological backgrounds that views social interaction as a key mechanism underlying research use. We assume that patients/clients and their health outcomes should be the primary focus of research use, as such patients/clients play a key role in all aspects of the process. We assume that the research evidence used has been ethically derived and that research use projects are ethically sound. A final assumption is that both the external or societal environment will affect all aspects of the process and must also be considered.

Background and context

Being aware of the lack of practical models to promote research use, we began assembling diverse aspects of the process into a simple and

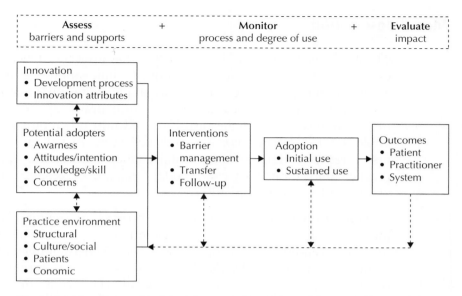

Figure 4.1 The Ottawa Model of Research Use (adapted from Graham and Logan, 2004, reproduced with permission)

useful framework. This we called the Ottawa Model of Research Use because we were both based in Ottawa, Canada and there was much work directed to transferring research into practice both in the hospital setting and in the research units with which we were associated. The model is informed by research, theory, and expert opinion. The elements of OMRU were supported by the available literature related to research utilization, the diffusion of innovations, health behavior change, and the development and implementation of practice guidelines (Logan and Graham, 1998). We also engaged in a process of reflection on our experience researching and practicing in the field, as well as, information gained through discussion with workshop participants, academic presentations, and clinical education rounds. The model was used for the first time and refined subsequently during an implementation project that was part of a province wide initiative to strengthen nursing professional practice (Logan *et al.*, 1999; Royle *et al.*, 2000). As research on knowledge use increased, so our ideas changed, and while keeping the original six elements as posited in 1998, we added or moved a number of subelements seen as important to successful implementation of research findings. Changes have focused on expanding important details within each element. The model diagram was altered accordingly (Fig. 4.1).

Model description

The model is comprised of six elements that are central to the process of research use: the research-informed innovation, the potential adopters, the practice environment, implementation interventions for transferring the research findings into practice, the adoption of the innovation, and the health-related and other outcomes (see Table 4.1 for definitions). Research continues to validate that the first three essential or fundamental elements affect the uptake of practice innovations (Foy *et al.*, 2002; Graham, 1998; Graham *et al.*, 2004; Grol and Wensing, 2004).

The prescriptive part of the model is a process of assessing, monitoring, and evaluating (AME). During the planning and implementing of a research-informed project using the OMRU, implementation facilitators are guided by the AME process prior to, during, and as the final steps of the project are completed. The facilitation role may be filled by a researcher, policy maker, administrator, educator, or a knowledgeable practitioner. Usually a team of individuals with different expertise is assembled to implement the innovation. Our 2004 version of the model provided a description of how to use the model (Graham and Logan, 2004a).

The innovation

The innovation represents something new to those who will use it (Rogers, 1995, 2003) and should be informed by valid research findings. It must be combined with the judgment of users. Research findings on health topics are often translated into various knowledge tools and products that form the research-informed innovation. It may be in the form of a policy, procedure, practice guideline, or similar vehicle (e.g., meta-analysis of quantitative studies or meta-synthesis of qualitative work). For consistency and to spare the introduction of numerous examples, we will use practice guidelines as an exemplar of a research-informed innovation throughout the remainder of the chapter. The selection of practice guidelines as the example is not intended to privilege this form of knowledge tool over others but much research has been conducted with practice guidelines as the focus.

In 2004 (Graham and Logan, 2004a) we changed the OMRU 1998 figure by placing the innovation box at the figure's top rather than at the bottom of the three fundamental elements, although individuals

Table 4.1 Definitions used in the Ottawa Model of Research Use

Concept	Definition
Adapting an innovation	Shaping a generic research-informed product (e.g., a practice guideline, policy, etc.) to a particular context to ensure a fit with other aspects of practice and with practitioner values. This must be done without disregarding the research evidence.
Adoption	Decision and action sequences by potential adopters including forming an intention to use, trying the innovation, continuing to use and adapting as necessary.
Attitudes	Potential adopter positive and/or negative stance about the innovation; position toward the change (general and specific to the innovation); opinions about the innovation.
Assessment profiles	A systematic delineation of the barriers and facilitators to the adoption of the innovation by the potential adopters in their practice setting.
Awareness	Potential adopter cognizance of the innovation.
Barrier management strategies	Strategies to actively manage any obstacles that could impede the uptake and use of the innovation.
Concerns	Potential adopter worries about or issues with the proposed innovation change.
Culture/social	Belief systems within the setting, local politics, personalities and leadership, peer influences, endorsement of the change by local champions.
Development process	Steps involved in reviewing the research that informs the innovation; creating and adapting the innovation.
Economic	Availability of resources, equipment, supplies necessary to implement and use the innovation.
Evaluation	Systematic determination of the consequences of using the innovation.
Facilitators	Individuals or groups who volunteer or are charged with responsibility for implementing the research-informed innovation.
Follow-up strategies	Actions taken to fix problems encountered during adoption and to assist potential adopters' use of the innovation.
Initial use	Potential adopters' actions when they first begin to use the innovation until their learning curve is completed.

(Continued)

Table 4.1 (*Continued*)

Concept	Definition
Innovation	A change that constitutes something new to those who will use it. It is informed by valid research and is combined with the clinical judgment of the practitioner. It may be in the form of a practice guideline, a policy, procedure, or similar vehicle.
Innovation attributes	Potential adopters' perceptions of the characteristics of the innovation (e.g., relative advantages, complexity, compatibility, clarity, user-friendliness).
Intention	Potential adopters decision to try the innovation in practice
Interventions	Passive or active actions to raise awareness, educate, persuade and facilitate adoption of the innovation. Specific strategies are tailored to the users and practice setting based on the assessment profiles.
Knowledge/skill	Information and skill potential adopters might have or need that could be required in the using/applying the innovation.
Monitoring	An ongoing process to determine the status of the barrier management and implementation strategies (e.g., are going as planned). It includes follow-up trouble shooting and contact with the potential adopters as they trial the innovation.
Outcome	Effects of using the innovation in practice following a successful implementation and adoption. Outcomes relate to the patient, practitioner, and system.
Patient/client	Patient, patient family, consumers, and others who should benefit from the innovation adoption.
Potential adopters	Practitioners, policy makers, or patients who may use or are involved in applying the innovation.
Practice environment	Setting in which the change in practice will occur.
Structure	Decision-making structure, rules, regulations, policies, physical structure of the setting, workload. Includes current practice: the existing/habitual way to provide care that the innovation adoption will change or affect.
Sustained use	Prolonged application of the innovation such that the desired outcomes might be expected to occur.
Tailoring	Modifying the implementation interventions to fit with the innovation, potential adopters, and the practice environment with the intent to increase adoption.
Transfer strategies	Facilitator actions taken to passively or actively get the necessary information and skill to the potential adopters.
Use	Potential adopters' application of the innovation in practice.

with different perspectives (i.e., scientist or practitioner) may wish to start a project with different elements, in almost all cases, when explaining or writing up a project, it is necessary to start with the innovation in order for subsequent discussion to make sense.

Guidelines (i.e., innovations) developed by credible sources using explicit and transparent processes including rigorous searching of the literature for research findings and incorporating objective methods to synthesize the evidence has been positively associated with guideline adoption (Logan and Graham, 1998). Involvement of end-users in developing innovations has also been reported to positively affect guideline adoption (Grol and Wensing 2005; Puech *et al.*, 1998) although this is not always the case (Silagy *et al.*, 2002; Wallin *et al.*, 2000). The potential adopters' perceptions of the attributes of the innovation have been shown to influence their decisions to adopt, use, or sustain their use (Rogers, 1995, 2003). Rogers (1995, 2003) noted that important innovation characteristics perceived by the potential adopters that affect the rate of innovation adoption include the relative advantage, compatibility, complexity, observability, and trialability. Specifically attributes positively related to guideline use include low complexity (i.e., easy to learn or use), compatibility with current practice or values and norms (i.e., do not require extensive change in current practice), high trialability (i.e., are easy to try out before committing to change), and guideline recommendations that are clear, noncontroversial, and evidence-based (Burgers *et al.*, 2003; Graham *et al.*, 2004; Grilli and Lomas, 1994; Grol and Wensing 2005; Grol *et al.*, 1998). In a pressured work environment, perceived advantage of the proposed innovation could be that associated costs would be less. We have found that complexity of a guideline is compounded when the issue is multidisciplinary, for example, if both physicians and nurses are essential to the practice (Graham *et al.*, 2004). As well complexity increases when the guideline requires two or more discrete types of actions, for example, one centered on technology and a second one on supportive care. Experience indicates that format and style of the guideline (i.e., user-friendly and attractive) play a part (Brown *et al.*, 1995).

The proliferation of practice guidelines on many topics has resulted in the need to choose among them carefully and to judge the quality of the guideline against rigorous standards (Graham *et al.*, 2003a). Selecting among synthesized evidence or several suitable practice guidelines also rests on feasibility issues and on the fit with current practice. Once selected, generic practice guidelines must be adapted to be compatible with the specific context. There is a useful model for the evaluation and adaptation of practice guidelines for local use (Graham *et al.*, 2002, 2003a, 2005) which has been validated (Harrison *et al.*, 2005).

Potential adopters

Practitioners, policy makers, or patients who may use the innovation are potential adopters. This element is comprised of: awareness, attitudes/intention, knowledge/skill, and concerns. We have revised the OMRU potential adopter element by adding three subelements. These include (a) awareness of the specific practice innovation; (b) intention to adopt; (c) concerns about the innovation. Awareness was added when it became clear that if potential adopters did not know of the innovation, there was no point assessing attitudes etc. Understanding the degree of awareness of the innovation and any misconceptions which will need clarification provides important information for planning implementation interventions. One way awareness can be heightened is by seeking feedback from potential adopters during the process to adapt the innovation to local circumstances. A systematic review on the individual determinants of research utilization by nurses confirmed the value of attitudes and information-seeking behavior (Estabrooks *et al.*, 2003). We moved the subelement "intention" to adopt the innovation from the adoption element to fit with attitudes because it represents the "decision" phase of Rogers (1995, 2003) five-phase adoption–innovation process (knowledge, persuasion, decision, implementation, confirmation). Our view now is that it is better seen as a predictor of adoption and therefore should be assessed with the other variables related to the potential adopter. Exploring intention to adopt provides information on barriers or facilitators to the adoption and thus to the intensity of the implementation interventions required. We added "concerns" as a subelement because even supportive potential adopters had concerns (e.g., about the patient outcomes, worry about added workload, etc.) that needed to be addressed. Concerns are potential adopter worries about or issues with the proposed innovation change. Considerable excellent work was done on this idea in the field of education by Hord *et al.* (1998) who outlined stages of concern in their concerns-based adoption model. We found concerns of potential adopters centered on potential outcomes for the patient if practice were changed and how the change would affect staff (Graham *et al.*, 2004). Associated with the prevailing worry that patient harm might occur was the subsequent concern over the threat of legal consequences (Graham *et al.*, 2004). A primary concern is frequently one of workload and the time involved to acquire the necessary skill and the time to carry out and sustain the new practice. Unaddressed concerns may become barriers to adoption.

Practice environment

The practice environment is comprised of structural factors that include decision-making structure, rules, regulations, policies, physical structure of the setting, workload, and current practice. Professional standards and medico-legal issues are important structural factors. The cultural/social factors include local politics, personalities, leadership, and peer opinion. Leadership plays an important role in many aspects of the practice environment (Gifford *et al.*, 2006). Patients and consumers who are involved with the health problem and the innovation are part of the practice environment as well as economic considerations regarding available resources. We have moved the subelement current practice to the practice environment element because it reveals the gap between how the care is being provided now and what is being recommended by the research and it provides information about potential barriers. We consider that the influence of peers is an important aspect of the overall cultural issues within the organization and practice setting (Graham *et al.*, 2004). A number of other factors related to the practice environment have been noted to affect adoption (Damanour, 1991; Estabrooks, 2003; Greenhalgh *et al.*, 2004).

With consideration of the three fundamental elements: the innovation, potential adopters, and practice environment, the OMRU prescriptive portion AME should begin. Understanding the three fundamental elements better enables problem solving, selection and tailoring of implementation interventions, and managing the implementation for adoption (initial and sustained use of the innovation), at which point evaluation of outcomes becomes possible.

Implementation interventions

We posit that interventions should be tailored to the specifics of the situation based on the assessment of the innovation, the potential adopters, and the practice environment. Because the existence of synthesized evidence does not ensure a change in practice, a variety of implementation interventions are necessary (Toman *et al.*, 2001).

The OMRU classifies interventions into three categories: barrier management strategies, passive and active implementation strategies, and follow-up activities. Barrier management strategies are intended to reduce or eliminate any identified barriers to adoption. Implementation strategies are aimed at transferring the research-informed innovation to the potential adopters and ensuring they have the needed skills to apply it. Follow-up strategies can identify any problems and assist potential adopters to sustain adoption. Interventions can vary in level of intensity from passive diffusion, targeted dissemination, to very active implementation strategies. Factors, such as the complexity of the innovation, the number of people involved (potential adopters), and their workload pressures (practice environment), complicate the situation. An innovation usually creates a potential adopter learning curve that requires follow-up interventions to ensure that the adopters have mastered the new activities. The follow-up determines if the innovation has been altered (reinvented or transformed) in some way that conflicts with the original evidence or that adopters have found the change impossible to do for any reason.

Research on the effectiveness of interventions to improve practice is increasing. The Cochrane Effective Practice and Organization of Care Group (EPOC) is a very good source of such evidence (http://www.epoc.uottawa.ca/reviews.htm). Others have summarized what is known about the effectiveness of implementation interventions (Bero *et al.*, 1998; Grimshaw *et al.*, 2004, 2006). Wensing *et al.* (2009) have recently provided a high-level review of reviews and presented the evidence for the effectiveness of many knowledge implementation interventions.

The general conclusions that can be drawn from the literature are that most interventions are effective under some circumstances but none are effective under all circumstances, hence the need to assess and monitor the specific situation. Few interventions have been well tested. Generalization from trials and systematic reviews of interventions is difficult because of the poor quality of the existing studies and poor understanding of the determinants of professional behavior change and barriers to research uptake. Furthermore, research into how to tailor interventions to barriers remains in its infancy (Bosch *et al.*, 2007). Therefore it is reasonable to suggest that when attempting to tailor the interventions to the identified barriers, facilitators should first consider interventions for which there is evidence of effectiveness but also be prepared to be flexible and experiment.

Adoption

We use the term adoption to mean action sequences by potential adopters including initially trying the innovation and continuing to use it. Adoption can take different forms. Here it becomes necessary explicate what constitutes knowledge use. The innovation is new knowledge to some or all of the potential adopters and their adoption of it is a form of "knowledge use." At least three types of knowledge use have been described (Beyer, 1997; Estabrooks, 1999) including: (a) conceptual use of knowledge which occurs from general enlightenment that increases understanding or changes attitudes; (b) instrumental use which is when knowledge is applied directly and is reflected in changes in behavior or practice; and (c) symbolic or strategic use in which the knowledge is used to legitimate and sustain predetermined positions. Instrumental use is of particular interest to achieve patient/client outcomes.

Initial use or sustained use of an innovation may vary among adopters based on their level of experience with the new practice and their degree of professional experience in general. We have modified the subelement "use" with the word initial. This period of initial use comprises the start of trying out the innovation until the learning curve is over and a degree of competence is achieved. We also rephrased subelement "sustainability" added in previous version (Graham and Logan, 2006) to "sustained use." The notion of sustained use is an important concern and reflects current research in this area (Davies and Edwards, 2009; Stacey *et al.*, 2006; Wallin *et al.*, 2003). Sustained or ongoing use is critical to achieving the expected outcomes and the factors influencing initial use may be quite different from those influencing sustained use.

Outcomes

Outcomes typically relate to patients, practitioners, and financial or system results. In the revised OMRU the focus of the outcome evaluation remains unchanged. We use the term outcome to mean the impact of implementing the innovation (i.e., the effect or outcome of adoption of the innovation as opposed to uptake or conformity of potential adopters to the innovation). Outcome evaluation should be tailored to the specific innovation recommendations and should be able to be determined a priori and use the most rigorous study design feasible. The final determination of outcomes should not occur before the learning curve of potential adopters is primarily completed.

Assessing, monitoring, and evaluating (AME)

Now that we have concluded a description of the six main elements of the OMRU, we will turn attention to the prescriptive AME process (see Table 4.2).

AME process no. 1 – assessing the innovation, potential adopters, and practice environment

The first step in the AME process is conducting an assessment of the three fundamental elements. The rationale is that research adoption is context specific hence the need for assessment. Assessments of the innovation, potential adopters, and the practice environment may be done sequentially or may proceed concurrently. Our guidance on how to conduct a barriers assessment is largely based on our research and experience. We have carried out assessments in a number of ways, including qualitative approaches involving interviewing a few key informants (relevant clinicians, managers, etc.) or conducting focus groups with those that will be affected by implementation of the innovation (Graham *et al.*, 2003b, 2004; Zitzelsberger *et al.*, 2004). Quantitative approaches have included surveying potential adopters (Brouwers *et al.*, 2004; Graham *et al.*, 2001, 2003c, 2007a–c; Légaré *et al.*, 2006, 2007). Depending on needs of the implementation project mixed methods are also useful for assessing barriers (Stacey *et al.*, 2005). Finally, we have conducted environmental scans, which have included chart audits and analysis of administrative databases (Friedberg *et al.*, 2002; Harrison *et al.*, 2001; Lorimer *et al.*, 2003). Légaré *et al.* (2008) and Gravel *et al.* (2006) have systematically reviewed health professionals' perceptions of barriers and facilitators to implementation of shared decision making and refined Cabana *et al.'s* (1999) framework for classifying practice guideline barriers and Espeland and Baerheim's (2003) modification of it. These works are useful starting points for thinking about the different types of barriers and supports that facilitators might wish to investigate in their barriers assessments. More recently Légaré (2009) has reviewed the concepts and conceptual models for assessing barriers and facilitators to knowledge use and some of the more quantitative assessment tools. Wensing and Grol (2005) also provide useful advice for undertaking barriers assessment and Estabrooks *et al.* (2002) provide measurement information within a Canadian context.

Table 4.2 AME: Assessing, monitoring, and evaluating

Focus	Purpose	Rationale
Assessing the innovation, potential adopters and practice environment		
Innovation Potential adopters Practice environment	(1) To develop a profile of those characteristics that will serve as either barriers or supports to integrating the innovation into practice, (2) to form the basis of a guide to selection and tailoring of implementation strategies.	(1) That perceptions of the attributes of the innovation and characteristics of the potential adopters and practice environment shape the rate of adoption of the innovation and that their influence may fluctuate overtime, (2) exposure to implementation strategies may change or modify the influences of how the innovation is perceived, potential adopters, and practice environment factors, (3) perceptions of the innovation and potential adopters' awareness, knowledge, skills, concerns, etc. may change with exposure to or personal experience with the innovation, (4) when barriers to research use have been identified, proactive implementation strategies can be mobilized to overcome them, (5) when supports are identified, these can be used to full advantage to bolster implementation efforts.
Monitoring implementation interventions and adoption		
Implementation strategies	(1) To ensure that no new barriers have emerged, (2) to determine if implementation strategies are working according to plan, (3) to identify if follow-up strategies need modifying.	(1) Monitoring of the intervention provides information about how well·barriers have been managed and if there is a need add new ones to address any new barriers (e.g., do they have sufficient equipment), (2) permits an assessment of the level or dose of the intervention received, (3) information can be used to modify the existing interventions, (4) follow-up activities in the setting can be a big aid with finding answers about the potential adopters experience trying out the innovation (e.g., do they know enough, etc.).

(Continued)

Table 4.2 (*Continued*)

Focus	Purpose	Rationale
Adoption	(1) Identify the type and degree of use by adopters.	(1) Outcomes cannot be accurately evaluated until correct application of the innovation by the majority of potential adopters in ensured, (2) information can be used to understand effectiveness of the implementation strategies.
Evaluating outcomes		
Outcomes	(1) To identify the impact of the adoption on outcomes, (2) to determine whether the efforts to promote the innovation adoption were worth it, (3) to ensure that professional standards of practice are met.	(1) Patient care and safety are critical aspects of health care and any change in practice is expected to be at least as safe and effective as the prior one, (2) required resources of time and money may be extensive in most research-informed projects, thus the benefit:cost ratio is important, (3) professional standards and medico-legal issues cannot be compromised by the implementation of an research-informed innovation.

AME process 2 – monitoring implementation interventions and adoption

Ongoing monitoring the process and degree of use following the implementation interventions is necessary. The dynamic nature of the process means changes occur during the project that may influence the uptake of the innovation, therefore need monitoring. Approaches to monitoring any changes to the three fundamental elements, the implementation interventions and the degree of use or adoption can be qualitative and/or quantitative and should be conceptualized as process of formative evaluation rather than summative evaluation. Many of the methods mentioned in the above section are appropriate here. The intent is to help understand what is happening so as to be able to make corrections to the implementation plan as required. After a suitable time for the potential adopters' acquisition of the necessary skills and to overcome other implementation problems, an evaluation is made of the outcomes.

AME process 3 – evaluating outcomes

Evaluating the impact of the innovation can be done using quantitative and qualitative designs and can include, for example, using surveys, chart audits, analysis of administrative databases, economic analysis, as well as interviewing patients, providers, and administrators about their perceptions of the impact of implementing the innovation. In some of our work, for example, we used healing rates, health-related quality of life, and supply costs as outcome indicators for an implementation study of evidence-based leg ulcer care (Harrison *et al.*, 2005). Being able to identify unintended consequences is also critical. Straus *et al.* (2009) explain the importance of measuring outcomes and provide guidance on how to go about doing it. Sheppard (2009) provides a framework for evaluating complex interventions and other authors (Bhattacheryya and Zwarenstein, 2009) also provide information. Kenny *et al.* (2009) describe economic evaluations of implementation interventions. Grol *et al.* (2004) also have several chapters on evaluation that present different study designs.

Intended audience/users

The OMRU may be applied at any level in the delivery of care (e.g., individual or team), organizational (unit, department, hospital), or health care system. The AME portion of the OMRU is of particular use to those in practice settings, while the structural portion of the model's six elements can provide a basis to other scientists in their work (Dredger *et al.*, 2007; Kazanjian and Howett, 2008; O'Donnell *et al.*, 2005; Tetroe *et al.*, 2008). The OMRU has appealed to those who work in quality improvement (McDonald *et al.*, 2004) because while not explicitly linked to Donabedian's (1988) germinal work describing health care quality production in terms of structure, process, and outcomes, the model captures these characteristics in addition to being research-informed.

Hypotheses and research possibilities

A central hypothesis of the OMRU is that selecting strategies that align with information gained from assessing the specific innovation, potential adopters, and practice environment will increase adoption of the innovation. As well, adoption of the innovation will increase when barriers to adoption have been addressed and/or reduced. The OMRU can be used to guide studies in which adoption is the dependent variable. For example, issues to be examined include the speed of adoption, the degree of adoption (e.g., the percentage who adopted), or how well the innovation was adopted (i.e., the fidelity to the innovation). Adoption could be considered an independent or a moderating variable in a study interested in the outcomes of the adoption. Multiple regression modeling would be useful for determining relationships and importance between and among the elements. Determining what type of tailored interventions work for whom is a critical area of potential work, and trials that examine follow-up strategies with no follow-up may lead to information about this area which we consider important.

Qualitative research questions surrounding the innovation, potential adopter, and practice environment elements and subelements within them may be useful in an attempt to expand and refine the definitions and add to knowledge about the importance of each subelement to adoption of the innovation. Relationships between and among the three fundamental elements could be examined. Qualitative methods using the OMRU are very suitable to explain why a quality implementation project failed or succeeded and for research studies that yielded unusual findings (Graham *et al.*, 2004).

We have used the OMRU in our own research both to guide the studies and as a frame to analyze data (Graham *et al.*, 2003b, 2004, 2007b; Harrison *et al.*, 2007). Other investigators have used the OMRU in a similar manner with their work (Légaré *et al.*, 2006; Santesso and Tugwell, 2008; Stacey *et al.*, 2005, 2008). The cited research was conducted using quantitative, qualitative, and mixed method designs and took place in many different types of settings. We refer the reader to the original studies for more details.

Critique (strengths and limitations of OMRU)

Strengths of the OMRU became clearer as it was used with health professionals from practice, policy, and research (Table 4.3). We have received positive feedback from those using the model that it is intuitive, reflects practice, and is very useful for complex projects.

One of the OMRU limitations is the model has not had as much evaluation as some other models, however, that is changing as researchers

Table 4.3 Strengths of the Ottawa Model of Research Use

1. Breaks down a fairly complicated social and scientific process into discrete achievable phases while providing an overview of the process.
2. Structures the process to include all those involved including health consumers.
3. Promotes adoption of the best research-informed recommendations after consideration of local circumstances.
4. Reduces the barriers to implementation as a result of enhanced buy-in from the participating stakeholders and tailoring of implementation interventions.
5. Useful for different health care professions as well as multidisciplinary/ interdisciplinary groups by providing a neutral common language frame.
6. Ensures that the process is transparent and reproducible.
7. Rigorous and systematic.

and practitioners become aware of the model and see its potential. Some have critiqued the OMRU as a linear process model. Although presented as a linear diagram (Fig. 4.1), the nature of the process should not be interpreted as unidirectional; the elements, when taken together represent an open system where all the model elements influence each other in ways that may not be completely predicted in advance. Most quality practice projects, like research projects, have a logical starting and finishing point despite the reality of implementation which is not without set backs and the need for reinforcing steps etc.

Implementation of the OMRU

The OMRU has evolved from lessons gained by using the model in practice settings (Graham *et al.*, 2004; Logan *et al.*, 1999). The model was useful to keep a complex project to implement a skin care program in a large surgical program of a tertiary care hospital on track (Graham and Logan, 2004b). As well, knowledge was gained as graduate students attempted to apply the OMRU in clinical projects, for example, the OMRU guided a pilot project with a neonatal transport team trying out a family assessment guide (Hogan and Logan, 2004). One barrier occurred when explanation of the OMRU to potential adopters was attempted at the same time as initially explaining the research-informed project. We recommend only discussing the OMRU model with the implementation facilitators who will be using it to guide the project. The exception, of course, is if specific potential adopters request the information. Usually potential adopters have sufficient learning about the innovation, implementation interventions, etc., therefore the OMRU explanations unnecessarily complicate the issue. Another barrier is for first-time student users, who have commented that it is complex and therefore time-consuming. Conversely, repeated use of the model facilitates efforts. While increasing, it is difficult to know the extent of the model use. We have been at professional conferences and found poster and paper presentations outlining OMRU implementation of which we were unaware. The OMRU is being used to address clinical problems that have been identified and prioritized within the region, for example, stroke and geriatrics (A. Fisher, APN Stroke, pers. comm.). As well, to achieve research-informed practice, the nursing department of an Ottawa teaching hospital (R. van den Berg, pers. comm.) uses the OMRU in their quality initiatives combined with the best practice guidelines of the Registered Nurses Association of Ontario (RNAO) (DiCenso *et al.*, 2003). OMRU has been used to implement guidelines for pain assessment and management (J. Bissonnette, pers. comm.). The model has also been used to implement pain guidelines in a children's hospital (Ellis *et al.*, 2007). OMRU was used in a dysphagia research project (R. Martino, pers. comm.). Doctoral theses have focused on introducing shared decision making into telenursing (Stacey, 2005) and into family practice (Légaré, 2005).

Future possibilities

While the OMRU is a practical model in specific contexts, paradoxically, we propose that it can be viewed as an ideal overarching framework that may encompass more specific and well-tested theories from other fields of learning relevant to the field of knowledge use. For example, more specific theories for developing or adapting innovations would fit under the OMRU construct for the research-based innovation. Theories such as those on organizational or on individual behavior would fit within the practice environment and potential adopter constructs respectively. Theories on learning or marketing could be situated within the intervention element to inform implementation strategies. Concurrently when the focus is on the AME portion of the model, theories related to assessment and evaluation could provide additional guidance. The resulting theoretical pluralism from embedding appropriate micro and mid-range theories within appropriate OMRU elements is suited particularly to research addressing complex issues in multiple environments. In such a situation the

OMRU may be used as the broad-based model to organize the required activities. Examples of specific, well-tested theories from other fields of learning that are appropriate for the enterprise have been encompassed within the OMRU generic constructs (Eccles *et al.*, 2006; McDonald *et al.*, 2004). Others have used the OMRU as a basis for their own theoretical possibilities (Kontos and Poland, 2009).

Conclusion

Getting research into practice requires a systematic effort on the part of many. The process is complex and occurs in the face of competing organizational and practice priorities. Therefore, researchers have an obligation to create, analyze and synthesize the theoretical and empirical underpinnings for practice change. Policy makers will achieve increased research use with clear and useful frameworks and theories to guide their efforts. The OMRU is proving to be a useful tool for policy makers, practitioners, and scientists to assist in their work. Armed with an understanding of the model with its strengths and limitations they are better equipped to select and apply an appropriate range of strategies when planning to implement change.

We aspire to present a framework for viewing research use that will be meaningful to scholars and useful to policy makers, practitioners, and implementation facilitators. The test of its meaningfulness and usefulness is not whether it accounts for everything that is happening in the research use field. Obviously it does not. The test is whether or not it provides a more meaningful and useful lens through which to view developments than alternatives (Kontos and Poland, 2009). We acknowledge that any lens is time-limited and that the field shifts overtime as more research becomes available.

Summary: How the model can be used/applied

- As a guide for evidence-based practice projects at agency or unit levels.
- As a guide for quality improvement projects.
- To provide a useful overview for multidisciplinary groups.
- To provide a design for implementation research projects.

- As a useful tool to frame data analysis for research projects focused on implementation or knowledge translation.
- As an overview model to imbed various specific theories pertinent to evidence-based projects, for example, learning theories, marketing theories.

References

Bero, L. A., Grilli, R., Grimshaw, J. M., Harvey, E., Oxman, A. D., and Thomas, M. A. (1998). Getting research findings into practice. Closing the gap between research and practice: An overview of systematic reviews of interventions to promote the implementation of research findings. *British Medical Journal*, 317, 465–468.

Beyer, J. M. (1997). Research utilization: Bridging the gap between communities. *Journal of Management Inquiry*, 6(1), 17–22.

Bhattacharyya, O. and Zwarenstein, M. (2009). The knowledge to action cycle: Methodologies to evaluate effectiveness of knowledge translation interventions. In: S. Straus, J. Tetroe, and I. D. Graham (eds), K*nowledge Translation in Health Care, Moving from Evidence to Practice*, Chapter 6a. Wiley-Blackwell: Oxford.

Bosch, M., Van der Weijden, T., Wensing, M., and Grol, R. (2007). Tailoring quality improvement interventions to identified barriers: A multiple case study analysis. *Journal Evaluation in Clinical Practice*, 13, 161–168.

Brouwers, M., Graham, I. D., Hanna, S. E., Cameron, D. A., and Browman, G. P. (2004). Clinicians' assessments of practice guidelines in oncology: The CAPGO survey. *International Journal of Technology Assessment in Health Care*, 20(4), 421–426.

Brown J. B., Shye, E., and McFarland, B. (1995). The paradox of guideline implementation: How AHCPR's depression guideline was adapted at Kaiser Permanente Northwest Region. *Joint Commission on Quality Improvement*, 21, 5–21.

Burgers, J. S., Grol, R. P., Zaat, J. O., Spies, T. H., van der Bij, A. K., and Mokkink, H. G. (2003). Characteristics of effective clinical guidelines for general practice. *British Journal General Practice*, 53(1), 15–19.

Cabana, M., Rand, C., Powe, N., *et al.* (1999). Why don't physicians follow clinical practice guidelines? A framework for improvement. *Journal of American Medical Association*, 282, 1458–1465.

Damanpour, F. (1991). Organizational innovation: A meta-analysis of effects of determinants and moderators. *Academy of Management Journal*, 34, 555–590.

Davies, B. and Edwards, N. (2009). The Action cycle: Sustaining knowledge use. In: S. Straus, J. Tetroe, and I. D. Graham (eds), K*nowledge Translation in Health Care, Moving from Evidence to Practice*, Chapter 3.6. Wiley-Blackwell: Oxford.

DiCenso, A., Bajnok, I., Virani, T., Borycki, E., Davies, B., Graham, I., *et al.* (2003). A toolkit to facilitate the implementation of clinical practice guidelines in health care settings. *Hospital Quarterly,* 5(3), 55–60.

Donabedian, A. (1988). The quality of care. How can it be assessed? *Journal of American Medical Association,* 260(12), 1743–1748.

Dredger, S. M., Kothari, A., Morrison, J., Sawada, M., Crighton, E. J., and Graham, I. D. (2007). Using participatory design to develop (public) health decision support systems through GIS. *International Journal of Health Geography,* November 27, 6, 53. PMID: 18042298 [PubMed – indexed for MEDLINE].

Eccles, M., Hanna, S., Logan, J., *et al.* (2006). Designing theoretically-informed implementation interventions. *Implementation Science.* Available at: http://www.implementationscience.com/content/pdf/1748-5908-1-4.pdf

Ellis, J., McCleary, L., Blouin, R., *et al.* (2007). Implementing best practice pain management in a pediatric hospital. *Journal of SPN,* 12(4), 264–277.

Espeland, A. A. and Baerheim, A. A. (2003). Factors affecting general practitioners' decisions about plain radiography for back pain: Implications for classification of guideline barriers – A qualitative study. *BMC Health Services Research,* March 24, 3, 8, doi: 10.1186/1472-6963-3-8. [PubMed].

Estabrooks, C. A. (1999). The conceptual structure of research utilization. *Research in Nursing and Health,* 22, 203–216.

Estabrooks, C. A. (2003). Translating research into practice: Implications for organizations and administrators. *Canadian Journal of Nursing Research,* 35(3), 53–68.

Estabrooks, C. A., Tourangeau, A., Humphrey, C. K., *et al.* (2002). Measuring the hospital practice environment: A Canadian context. *Research in Nursing & Health,* 25(4), 256–268.

Estabrooks, C. A., Floyd, J. A., Scott-Findlay, S., O'Leary, K. A., and Gushta, M. (2003). Individual determinants of research utilization: A systematic review. *Journal of Advanced Nursing,* 43, 506–520.

Foy, R., Penney, G., MacLennan, G., Grimshaw, J., Campbell, M., and Grol, R. (2002). Attributes of clinical recommendations that influence change in practice following audit and feedback. *Journal of Clinical Epidemiology,* 55, 717–722.

Friedberg, E., Harrison, M. B., and Graham, I. D. (2002). Current home care expenditures for persons with leg ulcers. *Journal of Wound Ostomy and Continence* Nursing, 29(4), 186–192.

Gifford, W. A., Davies, B., Edwards, N., and Graham, I. D. (2006). Leadership strategies to influence the use of clinical practice guidelines. *Nursing Leadership,* 19(4), 72–88.

Graham, I. D. (1998). Process of change in obstetrics: A cross-national case-study of episiotomy. *Health, An Interdisciplinary Journal for the Social Study of Health, Illness and Medicine,* 2, 403–433.

Graham, I. D. and Logan J. (2004a). Knowledge transfer and continuity of care research. *Canadian Journal of Nursing Research,* 36(2), 89–103.

Graham, K. and Logan, J. (2004b). Using the Ottawa Model of Research Use to implement a skin care program. *Journal of Nursing Care Quality*, 19(1), 18–24.

Graham, I. D. and Logan, J. (2006). How to influence medical practice: A conceptual framework. *Canadian Respiratory Journal*, 13(Suppl. A), 6A–7A.

Graham, I. D., Harrison, M. B., Moffat, C., and Franks, P. (2001). Leg ulcer care: Nursing attitudes and knowledge. *Canadian Nurse/L'Infirmiere Canadienne*, 97(3), 19–24.

Graham, I. D., Harrison, M. B., Brouwers, M., Davies, B., and Dunn, S. (2002). Facilitating the use of evidence in practice: Evaluating and adapting clinical practice guidelines for local use by health care organizations. *Journal of Obstetric, Gynecological, and Neonatal nursing*, 31, 599–611.

Graham, I. D., Harrison, M. B., and Brouwers, M. (2003a). Evaluating and adapting practice guidelines for local use: A conceptual framework. In: S. Pickering and J. Thompson (eds), *Clinical Governance and Best Value: Meeting the Modernization Agenda* (pp. 213–229). Churchill Livingstone: London.

Graham, I. D., Logan, J., O'Connor, A., *et al.* (2003b). A qualitative study of physicians' perceptions of three decision aids. *Patient Education and Counseling*, 50, 279–283.

Graham, I. D., Harrison, M. B., Shafey, M., and Keist, D. (2003c). Knowledge and attitudes regarding care of leg ulcers: Survey of family physicians. *Canadian Family Physician*, 49, 896–902.

Graham, I. D., Logan, J., Davies, B., and Nimrod, C. (2004). Transfer and uptake of national clinical practice guidelines on fetal health surveillance: A case study. Birth, 31(4), 293–301.

Graham, I. D., Harrison, M. B., Lorimer, K., *et al.* (2005). Adapting national and international leg ulcer practice guidelines for local use: The Ontario leg ulcer community care protocol. *Advances in Skin and Wound Care*, 18(6), 307–318.

Graham, I. D., Jette, N., Tetroe, J., Robinson, N., Milne, S., and Mitchell, S. L. (2007a). Oral Cobalamin remains medicine's best kept secret. *Archives of Gerontology and Geriatrics*, 44(1), 49–59.

Graham, I. D., Logan, J., Bennett, C. L., *et al.* (2007b). Physicians' intentions and use of three patient decision aids. *BMC Medical Informatics and Decision Making*, 7, 20. Available at: http://www.biomedcentral.com/1472-6947/7/20

Graham, I. D., Brouwers, M., Davies, C., and Tetroe, J. (2007c). Ontario doctors' attitudes toward and use of clinical practice guidelines in oncology. *Journal Evaluation of Clinical Practice*, 13(4), 607–615.

Gravel, K., Légaré, F., and Graham, I. D. (2006). Barriers and facilitators to implementing shared decision-making in clinical practice: A systematic review of health professionals' perceptions. *Implementation Science*, August, 1(16). Available at: http://www.implementationscience.com/content/1/1/16

Greenhalgh, T., Robert, G., Macfarlane, F., Bate, P., and Kyriakidou, O. (2004). Diffusion of innovations in service organizations: Systematic review and recommendations. *Milbank Quarterly*, 82(4), 581–629.

Grilli, R. and Lomas, J. (1994). Evaluating the message: The relationship between compliance rate and the subject of a practice guideline. *Medical Care*, 32(3), 202–213.

Grimshaw, J. M., Thomas, R. E., MacLennan, G., Fraser, C., Ramsay, C. R., Vale, L., *et al.* (2004). Effectiveness and efficiency of guideline dissemination and implementation strategies. *Health Technology Assessment*, 8(6), iii–iv, 1–72. Available at: http://www.ncchta.org/project.asp?PjtId=994

Grimshaw, J., Eccles, M., Thomas, R., *et al.* (2006). Toward evidence-based quality improvement. Evidence (and its limitations) of the effectiveness of guideline dissemination and implementation strategies 1966–1998. *Journal General Internal Medicine*, February 21 (Suppl. 2), S14–S20.

Grol, R. and Wensing, M. (2004). What drives change? Barriers to and incentives for achieving evidence-based practice. *Medical Journal Australia, 180*, S57–S60.

Grol, R. and Wensing, M. (2005). Characteristics of successful innovations. In: R. Grol, M. Wensing, and M. Eccles (eds), *Improving Patient Care. The Implementation of Change in Clinical Practice* (pp. 60–70). Elsevier: London.

Grol, R., Dalhuijsen, J., Thomas, S., Veld, C., Rutten, G., and Mokkink, H. (1998). Attributes of clinical guidelines that influence use of guidelines in general practice: Observational study. *British Medical Journal*, 317, 858–861.

Grol, R., Wensing, M., and Eccles, M. (2004). *Improving patient care. The implementation of change in clinical practice*. Elsevier: Toronto.

Harrison, M. B., Graham, I. D., Friedberg, E., Lorimer, K., and Vandevelde-Coke. S. (2001). Regional planning study. Assessing the population with leg and foot ulcers. *Canadian Nurse/L'Infirmiere Canadienne*, 97(2), 18–23.

Harrison, M. B., Graham, I.D., Lorimer, K., Friedberg, E., Pierschianowski. T., and Brandys, T. (2005). Leg-ulcer care in the community, before and after implementation of an evidence-based service. *Canadian Medical Association Journal*, 172, 1447–1452. Available at: http://www.cmaj.ca/cgi/content/full/172/11/1447

Harrison, M. B., Graham, I. D., Logan, J., Toman, C., and Friedberg, E. (2007). Evidence to practice: Pre-post implementation study of a patient/provider resource for self-management with heart failure. *International Journal of Evidence-Based Health Care*, 5(1), 92–101.

Hogan, D. and Logan, J. (2004). The Ottawa Model of Research Use: A guide to clinical innovation in the NICU. *Clinical Nurse Specialist Journal*, 18(5), 1–7.

Hord, S., Rutherford, W., Huling-Austin, L., and Hall. G. (1998). *Taking Charge of Change*. Southwest Educational Development Laboratory: Austin, TX.

Kazanjian, A. and Howett, C. (2008). A knowledge exchange model for supportive cancer care. Final Report to: Cancer Journey Action Group The Canadian Partnership Against Cancer, December. School of Population and Public Health, University of British Columbia: Vancouver.

Kenny, D. J., Cornelissen, E., and Mitton C. (2009). Economic evaluation of knowledge to action interventions. In: S. Straus, J. Tetroe, and I. D. Graham (eds), *Knowledge Translation in Health Care, Moving from Evidence to Practice*, Chapter 6b. Wiley-Blackwell: Oxford.

Kontos, P. C. and Poland, B. D. (2009). Mapping new theoretical and methodological terrain for knowledge translation: Contributions from critical realism and the arts. *Implementation Science*, 4(1), doi: 10.1186/1748-5908-4-1.

Légaré, F. (2005). Implementation of the Ottawa decision support framework in five family practice teaching units: An exploratory trial. PhD Dissertation, University of Ottawa.

Légaré, F. (2009). The knowledge to action cycle: Assessing barriers and facilitators to knowledge use. In: S. Straus, J. Tetroe, and I. D. Graham (eds), *Knowledge Translation in Health Care, Moving from Evidence to Practice*, Chapter 3.3. Wiley-Blackwell: Oxford.

Légaré, F., O'Connor, A. M., Graham, I. D., *et al.* (2006). Primary health care professionals' views on barriers and facilitators to the implementation of the Ottawa Decision Support Framework in practice. *Patient Education and Counseling*, November, 63, 380–390.

Légaré, F., Graham, I. D., O'Connor, A. M., *et al.* (2007). Prediction of health professionals' intention to screen for decisional conflict in clinical practice. *Health Expectations*, 10(4), 364–379.

Légaré, F., Ratté, S., Gravel, K., and Graham, I. D. (2008). Barriers and facilitators to implementing shared decision-making in clinical practice: Update of a systematic review of health professionals' perceptions. *Patient Education and Counseling,* 73(3), 526–535.

Logan, J. and Graham, I. D. (1998). Toward a comprehensive interdisciplinary model of health care research use. *Science Communication*, 20, 227–246.

Logan, J., Harrison M. B., Graham, I., Dunn, K., and Bissonette J. (1999). Evidence-based ulcer practice: The Ottawa Model of Research Use. *Canadian Journal of Nursing Research*, 31(1), 37–52.

Lorimer, K., Harrison, M. B., Graham, I. D., Friedberg, E., and Davies, B. (2003). Assessing venous leg ulcer population characteristics and practices in a home care community. *Ostomy Wound Management*, 49(5), 32–43.

McDonald, K. M., Graham, I. D., and Grimshaw, J. (2004). Toward a theoretic basis for quality improvement interventions. In: K. G. Shojania, K. M. McDonald, R. R. Wachter, and D. K. Owens (eds), *Closing the*

Quality Gap: A Critical Analysis of Quality Improvement Strategies: Volume 1 – Series Overview and Methodology, Chapter 3. Technical Review, 9(1). AHRQ, U.S. Department of Health and Human Services: Rockville, MD.

O'Donnell, S., Cranney, A., Jacobsen, M. J., Graham, I. D., O'Connor, A. M., and Tugwell, P. (2005). Understanding and overcoming the barriers of implementing patient decision aids in clinical practice. *Journal of Evaluation in Clinical Practice*, 12, 174–181.

Puech, M., Ward, J., Hirst, G., and Hughes, A-M. (1998). Local implementation of national guidelines on lower urinary tract symptoms: What do general practitioners in Sydney, Australia suggest will work? *International Journal for Quality in Health Care*, 10, 339–343.

Rogers, E. M. (1995). *Diffusion of innovations*, 4th edn. Free Press: New York.

Rogers, E. M. (2003). *Diffusion of innovations*, 5th edn. Free Press: New York.

Royle, J., Blythe, J., Ciliska, D., and Ing, D. (2000). The organizational environment and evidence-based nursing. *Nursing Leadership (CJNL)*, 13(1), 31–37.

Santesso, N. and Tugwell, P. (2008). Knowledge translation in developing countries. *Journal of Continuing Education in the Health Professions*, Winter, 26(1), 87–96.

Sheppard, S. (2009). The knowledge to action cycle: Monitoring knowledge use: Framework for evaluating complex interventions. In: S. Straus, J. Tetroe, and I. D. Graham (eds), *Knowledge Translation in Health Care, Moving from Evidence to Practice*, Chapter 3.5b. Wiley-Blackwell: Oxford.

Silagy, C. A., Weller, D. P., Lapsley, H., Middleton, P., Shelby-James, T., and Fazekas, B. (2002). The effectiveness of local adaptation of nationally produced clinical practice guidelines. *Family Practice*, 19(3), 223–230.

Stacey, D. (2005). Design and evaluation of an implementation intervention to enhance decision support by call centre nurses for callers facing values-sensitive health decisions. PhD Dissertation, University of Ottawa.

Stacey, D., Graham, I. D., O'Connor, A. M., and Pomey, M-P. (2005). Barriers and facilitators influencing call center nurses' decision support for callers facing values-sensitive decisions: A mixed methods study. *Worldviews on Evidence-Based Nursing*, 2(4), 184–195.

Stacey, D., Pomey, M-P., O'Connor, A., and Graham, I. D. (2006). Adoption and sustainability of decision support for patients facing health decisions: An implementation case study in nursing. *BMC Implementation Science*, 1, 17, doi: 10.1186/1748-5908-1-17. Available at: http://www.implementationscience.com/content/1/1/17 (24 Aug 2006).

Stacey, D., Chambers, S. K., Jacobsen, M. J., and Dunn, J. (2008). Overcoming barriers to cancer-helpline professionals providing decision support for callers: An implementation study. *Oncology Nursing Forum*, 35, 961–969.

Straus, S. E., Tetroe, J., Graham, I. D., Zwarenstein, M., and Bhattacharyya, O. (2009). The knowledge to action cycle: Monitoring knowledge use and evaluating outcomes of knowledge use. In: S. Straus, J. Tetroe, and I. D. Graham (eds), *Knowledge Translation in Health Care, Moving from Evidence to Practice*, Chapter 3.5a. Wiley-Blackwell: Oxford.

Tetroe, J., Graham, I. D., Foy, R., *et al.* (2008). Health research funding agencies' support and promotion of knowledge translation: An international study. *Milbank Quarterly, 86(1)*, 125–155.

Toman, C., Harrison, M. B., and Logan, J. (2001). Clinical practice guidelines: Necessary but not sufficient for evidence-based patient education and counseling. *Patient Education and Counseling, 42*, 279–287.

Wallin, L., Boström, A.-M., Harvey, G., Wikblad, K., and Ewald, U. (2000). National guidelines for Swedish neonatal care. Evaluation of the clinical application. *International Journal for Quality in Health Care, 12*, 465–474.

Wallin, L., Boström, A.-M., Wikblad, K., and Ewald, U. (2003). Sustainability in changing clinical practice promotes evidence-based nursing care. *Journal of Advanced Nursing, 41*, 509–518.

Wensing, M. and Grol, R. (2005). Methods to identify implementation problems. In: R. Grol, M. Wensing, and M. Eccles (eds), *Improving Patient Care. The Implementation of Change in Clinical Practice* (pp. 109–120). Elsevier: London.

Wensing, M., Bosch, M., and Grol, R. (2009). The knowledge to action cycle: Selecting, tailoring and implementing knowledge translation interventions. In: S. Straus, J. Tetroe, and I. D. Graham (eds), *Knowledge Translation in Health Care, Moving from Evidence to Practice*, Chapter 3.4a. Wiley-Blackwell: Oxford.

Zitzelsberger, L., Grunfeld, E., and Graham I. (2004). Family physician perspectives on practice guidelines related to cancer control. *BMC Family Practice, 5*, 25. Available at: http://www.biomedcentral.com/1471-2296/5/25

Chapter 5

Promoting Action on Research Implementation in Health Services (PARIHS)

Jo Rycroft-Malone

Key learning points

- The Promoting Action on Research Implementation in Health Services (PARIHS) framework was developed inductively and has been subsequently refined over time.
- Successful implementation is represented as a function of the nature of *evidence*, the quality of the *context* of implementation, and appropriate approaches to *facilitation*.
- The development of the framework has been robust and systematic, and as a result PARIHS appears to have good construct and face validity, therefore we are reasonably confident that PARIHS is a conceptually robust framework.
- The PARIHS framework should be useful for those wanting to implement evidence into practice, as well as those who are researching implementation.

Background

Originally conceived through a collaboration between Kitson *et al.* (1998), the Promoting Action on Research Implementation in Health Services (PARIHS) framework has been evolving and developing for over a decade (Harvey *et al.*, 2002; Kitson *et al.*, 2008; McCormack *et al.*, 2002; Rycroft-Malone, 2004; Rycroft-Malone *et al.*, 2002, 2004a, b). This chapter provides an overview of the framework, a consideration about how it has, and could be used and by whom, a critique of perceived strengths and weaknesses and plans for PARIHS' future use and development

Purpose and assumptions

PARIHS was conceived and developed as a means of understanding the complexities involved in the successful implementation (SI) of evidence into practice. It serves as both a practical and conceptual heuristic to guide and evaluate research implementation and practice improvement endeavors. As PARIHS is currently presented as a conceptual, rather than a process-orientated framework, although the inclusion of "facilitation" as one of its core concepts indicates that process is a necessary implementation ingredient. PARIHS maps out the elements that need attention before, during, and after implementation efforts. It is not yet described as theoretical framework, because there is still much to learn about the linkages between the concepts, elements, and subelement in the framework, which will be determined through further testing and development.

Arguably to date the prevalent view about theory and knowledge translation has tended to focus on positivistic interpretations that privilege cause and effect explanations, that is, if you do x then y will happen (Rycroft-Malone, 2007). PARIHS has not been explicitly aligned with one particular theoretical position or perspective; it could be populated by multiple theories, at multiple levels (Kitson *et al.*, 2008). However, despite the potential of the framework to be a theory container and/or guide, its development has been informed by Diffusion of Innovations theory, various organizational theories, and humanism.

The title of the framework privileges the implementation of *research* evidence in health services. On further reading it will become clear that evidence is conceived more broadly than just research, that is, it is acknowledged that decision making and service delivery are informed by more than research evidence. Despite this broad conception, an implicit assumption of the framework is that the implementation of good quality, relevant research is likely to result in improved outcomes for patients and health services (Rycroft-Malone *et al.*, 2002).

Background to PARIHS' development

Kitson *et al.* (1998) stated that:

> Despite growing acknowledgement within the research community that the implementation of research into practice is a complex and messy task, conceptual models describing the process still tend to be unidimensional suggesting some linearity and logic (p. 149).

During the 1990s evidence-based medicine was the dominant paradigm, and this entailed a particular approach to encouraging the use of research evidence in practice. At this time (which to a certain extent persists today) the focus was on developing the skills and knowledge of individual practitioner's to appraise research and make rationale decisions based on research evidence. However, using research in practice is a complex process involving the interplay of factors influencing an individual's behavior, beyond that of being able to critically appraise research. This was the context in which PARIHS emerged.

With the commitment to the development and refinement of the framework over time, its content has evolved; currently the most up to date content can be found in Rycroft-Malone *et al.* (2004b). Table 5.1 provides an overview of the various stages of development of PARIHS, the following sections describe these in more detail.

Development

PARIHS developed inductively from the originators' experience as change agents and researchers. This collective wisdom led to the proposition that successful implementation (SI) a function (f) of the nature and type of evidence (E), the qualities of the context (C) in which the evidence is being introduced, and the way the process is facilitated (F); $SI = f(E,C,F)$ (Kitson *et al.*, 1998).

Table 5.1 Summary of PARIHS' stages of development

Phase	Activities and related publications
Development	• Retrospective and theoretical analysis of four case studies. • Development and publication of original framework. • Kitson *et al.* (1998)
Concept analysis	• Undertaken on the three core concepts of PARIHS: *evidence, context,* and *facilitation* using Morses' concept analysis approach (1996). • This resulted in changes to the way that facilitation was conceptualized, and some changes to the content of context. • Rycroft-Malone *et al.* (2002). • Harvey *et al.* (2002). • McCormack *et al.* (2002). • Rycroft-Malone *et al.* (2004b).
Empirical enquiry	• Case studies of evidence into practice projects to check out the content validity of PARIHS. • This resulted in the addition of local information to the concept of evidence, and some additions to context including fit with strategic priorities and resources. It also strengthened the rationale for the need of facilitation and/or a facilitative process. • Rycroft-Malone *et al.* (2004a).
Empirical testing	• Evaluating the impact of different types of facilitation (enabling and technical) on the implementation of recommendations for continence care: A process and outcome evaluation. • Funded by European Union Framework 7 involving centers in the UK and NI, Ireland, Sweden, and the Netherlands (2009–2013).
Development of tools	• Development of diagnostic and evaluative tools for use in research and practice. • Development of facilitation toolkits. • Some initial items for tools can be found in Kitson *et al.* (2008).

The three elements evidence, context, and facilitation, and their sub-elements were each positioned on a high–low continuum. Theoretical and retrospective analysis of four studies including research, quality improvement, and practice development work, led to the proposition that the most successful implementation occurs when evidence is scientifically robust and matches professional consensus and patients' preferences ("high" evidence), the context receptive to change with sympathetic cultures, strong leadership, and appropriate monitoring and feedback systems ("high" context), and, when there is appropriate facilitation of change with input from skilled external and internal facilitators ("high" facilitation).

At this time three-dimensional matrices were developed (1998: 153) to demonstrate various positions along the three dimensions and high–low continua. Theoretically, it was proposed that the ideal position in the framework would be where evidence, context, and facilitation are all high.

Since PARIHS' conception and publication in 1998, it has undergone research and development work and been open to the scrutiny of others, through, for example, workshops and presentations. As a result of these activities, the content of PARIHS and some of the dynamics between its elements has evolved and changed over time. The following sections describe these development processes.

Concept analyses and case studies

Following conception of the framework, the next stage of development involved concept analyses (Morse, 1995; Morse *et al.*, 1996) of each of the dimensions: evidence (Rycroft-Malone *et al.*, 2004b), context (McCormack *et al.*, 2002), and facilitation (Harvey *et al.*, 2002). The findings resulted in a refinement, addition to, and clarity of, the concepts as originally conceived in the 1998 version of the framework. Significantly the concept of facilitation changed as did the application of the dynamic high–low. These changes were summarized by Rycroft-Malone *et al.* (2002, and the above concept analysis papers) (see Fig. 5.1).

In parallel to the concept analysis phase, a small empirical study was conducted to check out PARIHS' content validity. Specifically it aimed to address the following questions:

- What factors do practitioners identify as the most important in enabling implementation of evidence into practice?
- What are the factors practitioners identify that mediate the implementation of evidence into practice?
- Do the concepts of evidence, context, and facilitation constitute the key elements of a framework for getting evidence into practice?

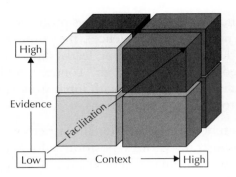

Figure 5.1 Evidence, context, facilitation

The study was conducted in two phases: (a) exploratory focus groups and (b) case studies of two sites with ongoing or recent implementation projects. The findings from this study resulted in additions to the concept of context, and in the addition of another subelement to evidence (local information/data). These findings and their impact on the framework are reported in Rycroft-Malone *et al.* (2004b).

The following sections describe the current versions of evidence, context, and facilitation (see Table 5.2 for content of each element) and therefore the most up to date version of the framework.

Evidence

Evidence is conceived in a broad sense within the framework including propositional and non-propositional knowledge from four different types of evidence: research, clinical experience, patients and carers' experience, and local context information (see Rycroft-Malone *et al.*, 2004b for a detailed discussion). For evidence to be located toward the "high" end of the continuum certain criteria have to be met, which are described in the following paragraphs.

Research evidence within PARIHS is only one part of the decision-making jigsaw, and indeed there are many issues where there is either a lack of research or the quality of it is poor. For research evidence to be situated at "high" on the continuum, whether it be qualitative and quantitative research, it should be well conceived and conducted, that is, robust and judged to be credible. Additionally evidence is socially and historically constructed and individuals and professionals will likely think differently about the same piece of

Table 5.2 PARIHS elements and subelements

Elements	Subelements		
Evidence		**Low**	**High**
	Research	• Poorly conceived, designed, and/or executed research • Seen as the only type of evidence • Not valued as evidence • Seen as certain	• Well conceived, designed, and executed research, appropriate to the research question • Seen as one part of a decision • Valued as evidence • Lack of certainty acknowledged • Social construction acknowledged • Judged as relevant • Importance weighted • Conclusions drawn
	Clinical experience	• Anecdote, with no critical reflection and judgment • Lack of consensus within similar groups • Not valued as evidence • Seen as the only type of evidence	• Clinical experience and expertise reflected upon, tested by individuals and groups • Consensus within similar groups • Valued as evidence • Seen as one part of the decision • Judged as relevant • Importance weighted • Conclusions drawn
	Patient experience	• Not valued as evidence • Patients not involved • Seen as the only type of evidence	• Valued as evidence • Multiple biographies used • Partnerships with health care professionals • Seen as one part of a decision • Judged as relevant • Importance weighted • Conclusions drawn

(Continued)

Table 5.2 (*Continued*)

Elements		Subelements	
	Local data/information	• Not valued as evidence • Lack of systematic methods for collection and analysis • Not reflected upon • No conclusions drawn	• Valued as evidence • Collected and analyzed systematically and rigorously • Evaluated and reflected upon • Conclusions drawn
Context		**Low**	**High**

	Culture	• Unclear values and beliefs
		• Low regard for individuals
		• Task-driven organization
		• Lack of consistency
		• Resources not allocated
		• Not integrated with strategic goals
			• Able to define culture(s) in terms of prevailing values/beliefs
			• Values individual staff and clients
			• Promotes leaning organization
			• Consistency of individuals role/experience to value:
			  – Relationship with others
			  – Teamwork
			  – Power and authority
			  – Rewards/recognition
			• Resources – human, financial, equipment – allocated
			• Initiative fits with strategic goals and is a key practice/patient issue

	Leadership	• Traditional, command, and control leadership • Lack of role clarity • Lack of teamwork • Poor organizational structures • Autocratic decision-making processes	• Transformational leadership • Role clarity • Effective teamwork • Effective organizational structures • Democratic inclusive decision-making processes

Table 5.2 (*Continued*)

Elements	Subelements		
	• Didactic approaches to learning/teaching/ managing	• Enabling/ empowering approach to teaching/learning/ managing	

Evaluation	• Absence of any form of feedback
	• Narrow use of performance information sources
	• Evaluations rely on single rather than multiple methods
		• Feedback on:
		  – Individual
		  – Team
		  – System performance
		• Use of multiple sources of information on performance
		• Use of multiple methods
		  – Clinical
		  – Performance
		  – Economic
		  – Experience evaluations	

Facilitation		**Low inappropriate facilitation**	**High appropriate facilitation**
	Purpose Role	Task Doing for others • Episodic contact • Practical/technical help • Didactic, traditional approach to teaching • External agents • Low intensity – extensive coverage	Holistic Enabling others • Sustained partnership • Developmental • Adult learning approach to teaching • Internal/external agents • High intensity – limited coverage
	Skills and attributes	Task/doing for others • Project management skills • Technical skills • Marketing skills • Subject/technical/ clinical credibility	Holistic/enabling others • Cocounselling • Critical reflection • Giving meaning • Flexibility of role • Realness/authenticity

research evidence (e.g., Dopson and Fitzgerald, 2005). Therefore to increase the likelihood of implementation, a process of appraisal and consensus development needs to take place so that it becomes valued as a valid part of the evidence base.

Evidence from clinical experience tempers research evidence; it is another strand of evidence. Clinical common sense needs to be evaluated to the same extent as research evidence. Therefore clinical experience needs to be made explicit and verified through critical reflection, critique, and debate with a wider community of practice to be considered at the high end of the continuum.

Evidence from patients is situated toward high when patients (and/or significant others) are part of the decision-making process during individual interactions and when patient narratives/stories are seen as a valid source of evidence.

Local information/data such as audit, performance, quality improvement, and evaluation information could be considered as part of the evidence base for practice if it has been systematically collected, evaluated, and reflected upon. If they meet these criteria local information/data would be considered "high."

PARIHS' conceptualization of evidence indicates the need for an interaction between the scientific and experiential through the blending of various types of information; this requires an interactive, participatory process guided by skilled facilitation.

Context

Context refers to the environment or setting in which the proposed change is to be implemented (see McCormack *et al.*, 2002 for a detailed discussion). Within PARIHS, the contextual factors that promote SI fall under three broad subelements: culture, leadership, and evaluation that operate in a dynamic, multileveled way.

Culture: Within PARIHS it is proposed that organizations that have cultures which could be described as "learning organizations" are those that are more conducive to change ("high"). Such cultures contain features such as decentralized decision making, a focus on relationships between managers and workers, and management styles that are facilitative.

Leadership: Leaders have a key role to play in creating such cultures. In PARIHS leadership summarizes the nature of human relationships in the practice context. In this sense leadership has the potential to bring about clear roles, effective teamwork, and effective organizational structures. Transformational leaders, as opposed to those that command and control, have the ability to create receptive contexts and challenge individuals and teams in an enabling, inspiring way ("high").

Evaluation: Contexts with evaluative mechanisms that collect multiple sources of evidence of performance that feedback at individual, team, and system levels comprise the third element of a "high" context. This is because such contexts not only accept and value different sources of feedback information but also create the conditions for practitioners to apply them into practice as a matter of course.

The context of practice is complex and dynamic. Specifically it is proposed that a conducive context for evidence-based practice is where there is clarity of roles, decentralized decision making, staff are valued, transformational leadership, and a reliance on multiple sources of information on performance.

Facilitation

Facilitation refers to the process of enabling or making easier the implementation of evidence into practice (see Harvey *et al.*, 2002 for a detailed discussion). Facilitation is achieved by an individual carrying out a specific role: a facilitator, with the appropriate skills and knowledge to help individuals, teams, and organizations apply evidence in practice. It is proposed that a facilitator has a key role to play in not only affecting the context of implementation but in working with practitioners to help them "make sense of" and apply evidence; and therefore is likely to be critical to the success or failure of implementation efforts.

Essentially the operationalization of the facilitator role will depend on the underlying purpose, stakeholders, nature of evidence, and context being worked with. Within PARIHS the purpose of facilitation can vary from being task orientated, which requires technical and practical support (e.g., administrating, taking on specific tasks), to enabling, which requires more of a developmental, process-orientated approach. It is argued that the skills and attributes required to fulfil the role are likely to depend on the situation, individuals, and contexts involved. Therefore skilled facilitators are those that can adjust their role and style to the different stages of an implementation project and the needs of those they are working with.

Testing

The development of the framework has been robust and systematic, and as a result PARIHS appears to have good construct and face validity (see the following section on its use by others), therefore we can be reasonably confident that PARIHS is a conceptually robust framework. However, it still needs further testing and scrutiny. We are now in the process of testing facilitation as conceived within PARIHS (Harvey *et al.*, 2002), in an intervention study. Funding was won to conduct a European multisite pragmatic process and outcome trial to evaluate two types of facilitation (technical and enabling). Technical and enabling facilitation approaches will be evaluated in comparison to each other and standard dissemination, for the implementation of continence recommendations for people over 60 in long-term care. This project started in January 2009 – and its progress can be followed at http://www.parihs.org. There remain many opportunities to test the framework in intervention studies.

Development of tools

As part of the development and testing phases of PARIHS, consideration has also been given to the development of tools that facilitate its practical application. For example, a number of questions were presented in our recent publication (Kitson *et al.*, 2008), which could be used in the diagnostic phase of an implementation study to identify what it is about evidence and context that needs attention from appropriate (i.e., "bespoke") facilitation interventions (see Table 5.3). Our intention is that these questions could be used by, for example, facilitators/leads/change agents to make a "diagnosis" of the situation, which will facilitate the planning of particularized and contextually appropriate interventions. Equally, these questions could be used to evaluate implementation efforts post hoc: what worked, what did not work, and why?

Intended users

Because PARIHS is a framework that represents the elements that play a potential role in the SI of evidence into practice, the intention is that it could be used by anyone either attempting to get evidence

Table 5.3 Diagnostic and evaluative questions

Evidence	Characteristics of evidence in the PARIHS framework (see Table 5.2)	Evidence: diagnostic/evaluative questions
Research		
	Well conceived, designed, and executed research appropriate to the research question	The research evidence is of sufficiently high quality
	Seen as one part of a decision	The research will be used as one part of the evidence
	Lack of certainty acknowledged	I value the research evidence
	Social construction acknowledged	The research evidence fits with my understanding of the issue
	Judged as relevant	The research evidence is useful in thinking about the issue
	Importance weighted	I am clear about what the key messages for the planned intervention are
	Conclusions drawn	There is consensus among my colleagues about the usefulness of this research to this issue
Clinical experience		
	Clinical experience and expertise reflected upon, tested by individuals and groups	I have reflected on my own clinical experience in relation to this issue
	Consensus within groups	I have shared and critically reviewed my clinical experience in relation to this issue
	Valued as evidence	I have shared and critically reviewed my clinical experience with knowledgeable colleagues outside of my (clinical) workplace
	Seen as one part of the decision	There is a consensus of (clinical) experience about this issue
	Judged as relevant	Clinical experience will be used as one part of the evidence
	Importance weighted	The consensus of clinical experience fits with my understanding of the issue
	Conclusions drawn	Clinical experience evidence is useful in thinking about the issue
		I am clear what the key messages for the planned intervention are

(Continued)

Table 5.3 *(Continued)*

Evidence	Characteristics of evidence in the PARIHS framework (see Table 5.2)	Evidence: diagnostic/evaluative questions
Patient experience		
	Valued as evidence	We routinely (and systematically) collect users/patients' experiences about this particular issue
	Multiple biographies used	Users/patients experiences will be used as one part of the evidence
	Partnerships with health care professionals	I value patient experiences evidence
	Seen as one part of a decision	The evidence of patients experiences fits my understanding of the issue(s)
	Importance weighed	Patient experiences are useful in thinking about the issue
	Conclusions drawn	I am clear about what the key messages for the planned intervention are
		There is a consensus among my colleagues about the usefulness of patient experiences to this issue
Information/data from local context		
	Valued as evidence	Data/information is routinely (and systematically) collected about this issue
	Collected and analyzed systematically and rigorously	Data/information from the local context will be used as one part of the evidence
	Evaluated and reflected upon	I value the data/information from the local context
	Conclusions drawn	The data/information from the local context fits with my understanding of the issue(s)
		The date/information from the local context is useful in thinking about the issue
		I am clear about what the key messages for the planned intervention are
		There is a consensus among my colleagues about the usefulness of the information/data from the local context for this issue

Table 5.3 *(Continued)*

Context	Characteristics of context in the PARIHS framework (seeTable 5.2)	Context: diagnostic/ evaluative questions
The environment or setting in which the proposed change is to be implemented		
Receptive context		
	Physical/social/cultural/structural/ system –boundaries clearly defined and acknowledged	The physical location is conducive to the implementation of this issue
	Professional/social networks clearly defined and acknowledged	There are sufficient human resources to implement this intervention successfully
	Appropriate and transparent decision-making processes	There are sufficient financial resources to implement this intervention successfully
	Power and authority processes	There is the right equipment to implement this intervention successfully
	Human/financial /technological/ equipment – resources appropriately allocated	There is the right IT support to implement this intervention successfully
	Information and feedback systems in place	I have access to the appropriate/useful professional networks and implement this intervention successfully
	Initiative fits with strategic goals and is seen as a key priority	The intervention fits with the strategic intent and goals of the organization
	Receptiveness/openness to change/ new ideas	Decision-making processes in the organization are clear to me

(Continued)

Table 5.3 *(Continued)*

Context	Characteristics of context in the PARIHS framework (see Table 5.2)	Context: diagnostic/evaluative questions
		I have the power and authority to carry out this intervention
		I have access to the appropriate skills and knowledge to carry out this intervention
Culture		
	Able to define culture(s) in terms of prevailing values/beliefs	This organization values innovation
	Values individual staff and clients	This organization values people who innovate
	Promotes learning of organization	This organization values staff as individuals
	Consistency of individual role/experience to value:	This organization values open communication and dialog
	• Relationships with others • Team work • Power and authority • Rewards/recognition	
		I feel there is open communication and dialog within my immediate work place
		I value open communication and dialog
		This organization values collaborative partnership working
		I feel there is collaborative partnership working in the wider organization
		I feel there is collaborative partnership working within my immediate work place
		I value collaborative partnership working
		There is a culture of continuous improvement in this organization
		There is a culture of continuous improvement with my immediate workplace
		This organization embraces change
		This organization values patients as individuals

Table 5.3 (*Continued*)

Context	Characteristics of context in the PARIHS framework (see Table 5.2)	Context: diagnostic/evaluative questions
Leadership		My immediate workplace embraces change
		This organization involved key stakeholders when introducing change
	Role clarity	I am clear what my role is within the team
	Effective teamwork	I am clear what my role is in the implementation of this initiative
	Effective organizational structures	I am clear what the lines of accountability are in terms of my role in implementing this initiative
	Democratic, inclusive decision making	I have been involved in determining how this initiative is going to be implemented
	Enabling/empowering approach to learning/ teaching/ managing	I have been able to develop new skills through this process
		I feel that I have learnt new skills and competencies
Evaluation	Feedback on individual/ team/system performance	We have routine mechanisms in place to collect data on
		• Individual performance (e.g., appraisal, clinical supervision, 360° feedback)
		• Team performance (e.g., audit and feedback, patient feedback, 360° feedback)
		• System performance (e.g., audit and feedback, formal inspections, economic data)
	Use of multiple sources of information on performance	Multiple sources of evaluation are used routinely in my workplace
	Use of multiple methods – clinical/individual/personal/ economic/patient experience	This type of evaluative information is routinely used to improve and change practice
	Range of routine measures collected by teams	The external data we collect is used by us to inform and improve our everyday practice.

into practice, or anyone who is researching or trying to better understand implementation processes and influences. Those who are actively attempting to implement evidence into practice could use the elements and subelements as a guide to what should be paid attention to in implementation projects. Researchers could use PARIHS as a theoretical framework, and as suggested above, a guide for developing interventions, and developing evaluative tools.

Hypotheses and propositions

Over the years the following working hypotheses have been presented:

- Most SI will occur when evidence is "high," practitioners agree about it, the context is developed, and where there is appropriate facilitation.
- Least SI occurs when context and facilitation are inadequate.
- Poor contexts can be overcome by appropriate facilitation.
- Chances of SI are still weak, even in an adequate context, but where there is inappropriate facilitation.

These are very broad hypotheses; however, the framework does offer the potential for more specific hypothesis development, particularly in relation to the potential for intervention research. The following are presented *as examples* of more specific (untested) hypotheses and also provide an illustration of the way that anyone could take the framework and develop their own relevant research questions and/or hypotheses.

- More enabling facilitation (holistic) approaches will be more effective at sustained practice improvement than technical (task) facilitation approaches.
- Feedback on individual and team performance (evaluation) using multiple sources of information will provide motivation for improvement.
- Developing a consensus about research evidence (evidence) among its users is more critical to implementation than developing a receptive context.
- Good teamwork (context) will determine the success of implementation.

- Particularizing facilitation approaches to the situation, people, and evidence will be more effective than using "off the shelf" interventions.
- Patient's experience (evidence) can be a more powerful lever of change than research evidence.

Others' use of PARIHS

As described in the earlier text the framework has good face and content validity, and has been included in reviews about knowledge translation (e.g., Greenhalgh *et al.*, 2004; Sudsawad, 2007) as well as individual studies and projects. Its face validity probably accounts for its growing use in implementation activities, evaluation, and research. A simple Google Scholar search using the term "PARIHS framework" yielded approximate 16,800 hits (performed March 12, 2009). Clearly this is a combination of citations (i.e., referencing PARIHS within evidence-based practice articles and presentations) and reports of its actual use or application (e.g., in practice, research, and/or evaluation).

Given the perceived extent of PARIHS' use, the following does not represent an exhaustive account, rather an illustration of use based on how, in a broad sense, it has been applied in others' work. This use appears to fall under three broad headings:

- as a conceptual/theoretical framework for research and evaluation;
- as the basis for tool development;
- for modeling research utilization.

Conceptual/theoretical framework for research and evaluation

Most commonly PARIHS has been used with research and implementation activity as a conceptual and theoretical framework, that is, as an organizing framework to underpin and/or guide implementation research and efforts (e.g., McSherry *et al.*, 2006; Sharp *et al.*, 2004). For example, Brown applied PARIHS to her research study in which pain management services were being developed (Brown and McCormack, 2005). In a review of the literature about the factors that have an influence on getting evidence into practice in post operative pain assessment and management, PARIHS was used an organizing framework to guide an analysis of the evidence. Using the main elements and subelements of the framework an exploration of the factors that might influence the successful development of an evidence-based pain management service were elicited under the broad headings evidence, context (including culture, leadership, and evaluation), and facilitation. These findings were then used as a guide to develop appropriate change strategies through action research and facilitation.

Ellis *et al.* (2005) provide another example of PARIHS being used as a conceptual framework. In this study the aims were to explore the relative and combined importance of context and facilitation in the implementation of a protocol and to establish individual and organizational change based on the principles of evidence-based practice. Ellis *et al.* used the PARIHS framework to facilitate the description of the processes and outcomes of an evidence-based practice training program delivered in Western Australia. It appears that the authors used evidence, context, and facilitation as a coding framework in the analysis of interview data, including the application of the high-to-low continuum to each element. The authors report that the PARIHS was helpful in explaining the outcomes of the education program.

Other examples of PARIHS being used as a conceptual framework include:

- Doran and Sidani (2007) who used the framework to develop and operationalize the development of an outcome focused knowledge translation intervention. In this example PARIHS was used to conceptualize the relationships among the factors that influence evidence-based nursing.
- Meijers *et al.* (2006) used the context element of the PARIHS framework to theoretically frame a systematic review of literature reporting the relationship between contextual factors and research utilization. In this example their review successfully mapped to the dimensions of context (culture and leadership), but not onto the subelement of evaluation.
- Wright *et al.* (2007) applied PARIHS within a study that evaluated the context within which continence care is provided in rehabilitation units for older people. They used the dimensions of context to direct data collection activities and the high–low continuum as a way of assessing the "state" or conduciveness of context for change.

- Conklin and Stolee (2008) used PARIHS to guide the evaluation of a health research transfer network and concluded that it had the potential to be used as a guide for evaluating other knowledge networks.
- Milner *et al.* (2006) used the "revised" PARIHS framework (Rycroft-Malone *et al.*, 2002) to inform the analysis of a systematic literature review of the research utilization behaviors of clinical nurse educators. Essentially they used the framework as a map to consider the sort of issues that were emerging from the review. They report their findings did not map onto the context variables in PARIHS, but did for the evidence and some of the facilitation elements.

Measurement

The other way that PARIHS has been used is as the basis for the development of measures or measurement tools. Two examples of PARIHS being used in this way are evident. McCormack *et al.* (2009) have developed a context assessment index (CAI), which links to PARIHS through examination of the three subelements in context: culture, leadership, and evaluation. A five-stage instrument development and testing approach was used to develop a psychometrically acceptable 37-item, 5-factor instrument. The purpose of this tool is to assist practitioners with assessing and understanding the context in which they work and the effect this has on implementing evidence into practice. The authors encourage others to use and further test the instrument in other settings and with different clinical topics.

Second, Estabrooks *et al.* (personal correspondence) have developed the Alberta Context Tool (ACT). This instrument includes items derived from the three subelements of context: culture, leadership, and evaluation. It was developed using appropriate psychometric processes, it has been designed to measure the context of research utilization, and has been tested in different settings with different groups of professionals. Similarly Helfrich *et al.* (2009) used the concepts of evidence, context, and facilitation from the PARIHS framework to develop an organizational readiness tool.

Modeling research utilization

Wallin *et al.* (2006), Estabrooks *et al.* (2007), and Cummings *et al.* (2007) report on a program of work that used the context element of PARIHS as the basis for developing a derived measure of research utilization, which was then used in multilevel modeling (structural equation modeling) to predict research utilization among nurses. While the elements of context were interpreted and applied by this team, which were different from the PARIHS team's conception of context (see Rycroft-Malone, 2007 for further critique, and McCormack *et al.*, 2002; Rycroft-Malone *et al.*, 2004b for concept analyses), their work supports the importance of contextual factors to research utilization. However the role of facilitation was less clear as a predictor of research use and they also point out that much of the variance in their modeling was accounted for by individual factors.

Critique (strengths and weaknesses) of PARIHS

There are a number of strengths and weaknesses related to PARIHS, which have been observed by others and the PARIHS team itself. The following outlines some of the questions that remain about PARIHS.

(1) How do the elements (evidence, context, and facilitation) and subelements interrelate and interact with each other and across different layers of the organization?
(2) Do the elements and subelements have equal weighting in getting evidence into practice?
(3) How does the individual practitioner fit into the framework?
(4) Is the content of the framework comprehensive?
(5) Is it greater than the sum of its parts?

Further empirical testing and evidence reviews of accumulated research may begin to determine some of the answers to these questions. Equally, it may be the case that because using evidence in practice is process orientated and contextually dependant, the answers to the interaction questions and those about weighting may not be answerable; that is, elements may interact and be weighted differently depending on the situation, people, and topic.

The question about how the individual fits into PARIHS is pertinent. Implicitly, individuals would be those that facilitators work with. Additionally practitioners' use of different sources of evidence in individual decision making is implicitly, not explicitly, represented within PARIHS. However, the role of the individual in decision making related to PARIHS has begun to be explored by Rycroft-Malone *et al.* (2009).

Equally, PARIHS has a number of strengths. Fundamentally it appears to have a high degree of face validity, that is, it accords with people's experiences of trying to implement evidence into practice, which probably accounts for its increasing use. Specifically, the strengths of PARIHS include the following.

- It is parsimonious with good content validity that facilitates guiding and evaluating implementation efforts.
- It provides both a broad, but if required specific, map of the factors that need to be considered for SI.
- It is flexible enough to be applied to a wide variety of topics, different clinical settings, patients, and professional groups.
- It can be populated by different theoretical approaches and theories, which means that it is amenable to use in studies using a variety of methodological approaches, which test, apply, and develop theory.

Future plans

Consistent with the commitment to continual refinement and development, there are plans to update the concept analyses of evidence, context, and facilitation. It is possible that this process will result in some changes to the subelements of PARIHS.

As a published framework, and as the preceding paragraphs have outlined, others have developed measurement tools, based on PARIHS' content. Generally, and naturally, these have been based on the developer's conceptions or interpretations of both the framework and the elements it contains. As part of a larger program of work within the European intervention project described earlier, measurement tool development work is planned. Further intervention work is planned and funding being sought.

A PARIHS international collaboration has also been created (http://www.parihs.org). The aim of the collaboration is to advance the development, testing, and refinement of PARIHS with a wide group of international stakeholders. The collaboration is a self-funded community that shares an interest in using and applying the PARIHS framework. Collaborative partners are individuals, teams, and/or organizations, who are willing to "sign up" to a number of ways of working principles.

Conclusion

The development of PARIHS has been a team effort and our various publications chart this journey. As a framework for implementing evidence into practice it appears to have good face validity and has been of use to others involved in implementation. The core elements – evidence, context, and facilitation have stood up to scrutiny, while the subelements have been subject to refinement and development. Our intention is to further develop the framework's utility, through the development of tools and resources. We also plan to test the hypotheses and propositions that PARIHS offers through intervention studies and development projects. Our hope is that we are able to do this development work in collaboration with a wider community, and encourage those interested in being involved in this endeavor to visit http://www.parihs.org

Summary: How PARIHS could be used

- PARIHS is a conceptual framework that represents the ingredients necessary for the successful implementation of evidence into practice. Therefore it could be used in diagnosis of readiness or in post-implementation evaluation.
- The PARIHS framework should be useful for those wanting to implement evidence into practice, as well as those who are researching implementation.
- The PARIHS framework has been used in a number of different ways, which broadly includes:
  - as a conceptual/theoretical framework for research and evaluation;
  - as the basis for tool development;
  - for modeling research utilization.
- The elements and subelements have been used to develop diagnostic and evaluative questions, which could guide implementers into developing particularized interventions.
- The framework offers the potential for hypothesis development, particularly in relation to the potential for intervention research.
- An international PARIHS collaboration has been developed which is a repository for how others have used the framework, and for the posting of any ongoing developments. This can be accessed at http://www.parihs.org.

References

Brown, D. and McCormack, B. (2005). Developing postoperative pain management: Utilising the Promoting Action on Research Implementation in Health Services (PARIHS) framework. *Worldviews on Evidence-based Nursing*, 2(3), 131–141.

Conklin, J. and Stolee, P. (2008). A model for evaluating knowledge exchange in a network context. *Canadian Journal of Nursing Research*, 40(2), 116–124.

Cummings, G.G., Estabrooks, C.A., Midodzi, W.K., Wallin, L., and Hayduk, L. (2007). Influence of organizational characteristics and context on research utilization. *Nursing Research Supplement*, 56(4S), S25–S39.

Dopson, S and Fitzgerald, L. (eds). (2005). *Knowledge to Action? Evidence-based Health Care in Context*. Oxford: Oxford University Press.

Doran, D. and Sidani, S. (2007). Outcomes-focused knowledge translation: A framework for knowledge translation and patient outcomes improvement. *Worldviews on Evidence-Based Nursing*, 4(1), 3–13.

Ellis, I., Howard, P., Larson, A., and Robertson, J. (2005). From workshop to work practice: An exploration of context and facilitation in the development of evidence-based practice. *Worldviews on Evidence-based Nursing*, 2(2), 84–93.

Estabrooks, C.A., Midodzi, W.K., Cummings, G.G., Wallin, L., and Adewale, A. (2007). Predicting research use in nursing organizations: A multi-level analysis. *Nursing Research Supplement*, 56(4S), S7–S23.

Greenhalgh, T., Robert, G., Bate, P., Kyriakidou, O., Macfarlane, F., and Peacock, R. (2004). *How to Spread Good Ideas. A Systematic Review of the Literature on Diffusion, Dissemination and Sustainability of Innovations in Health Service Delivery and Organisation*. London: National Co-ordinating Centre for NHS Service Delivery and Organisation. Available at: http://www.sdo.lshtm.ac.uk.

Harvey, G., Loftus-Hills, A., Rycroft-Malone, J., Titchen, A., Kitson, A., McCormack, B., and Seers, K. (2002). Getting evidence into practice: The role and function of facilitation . *Journal of Advanced Nursing*, 37(6), 577–588.

Helfrich, C.D., Yu-Fang, Li., Sharp, N.D., and Sales, A.E. (2009). Organizational readiness to change assessment (ORCA): Development of an instrument based on the Promoting Action on Research in Health Services (PARIHS) framework. *Implementation Science*, 4, 38 (accessed 14 July 2009).

Kitson, A.L., Harvey, G., and McCormack, B. (1998). Enabling the implementation of evidence-based practice: A conceptual framework. *Quality in Health Care*, 7(3), 149–158.

Kitson, A., Rycroft-Malone, J., Harvey, G., McCormack, B., Seers, K., and Titchen, A. (2008).Evaluating the successful implementation of evidence into practice using the PARIHS framework: Theoretical and practical challenges. *Implementation Science*, 3, 1 (accessed 7 January 2008).

McCormack, B., Kitson, A., Harvey, G., Rycroft-Malone, J., Titchen, A., and Seers, K. (2002). Getting evidence into practice – The meaning of 'context'. *Journal of Advanced Nursing*, 38(1), 94–104.

McCormack, B., McCarthy, G., Wright, J., Slater, P., and Coffey, A. (2009). Development and testing of the context assessment index (CAI). *Worldviews on Evidence-Based Nursing*, 6(1), 27–35.

McSherry, R., Artley, A., and Holloran, J. (2006). Research awareness: An important factor for evidence based practice. *Worldviews on Evidence-Based Nursing*, 3(3), 103–115.

Meijers, J.M.M., Janssen, M.A.P., Cummings, G., Wallin, L., Estabrooks, C.A., and Halfens, R.Y.G. (2006). Assessing the relationships between contextual factors and research utilisation in nursing: Systematic literature review. *Journal of Advanced Nursing*, 55(5), 622–635.

Milner, M., Estabrooks, C.A., and Myrick, F. (2006). Research utilization and clinical nurse educators: A systematic review. *Journal of Evaluation in Clinical Practice*, 12(6), 639–655.

Morse, J.M. (1995). Exploring the theoretical basis of nursing using advanced techniques of concept analysis. *Advances in Nursing Science*, 17, 31–46.

Morse, J.M., Hupcey, J.E., and Micham, C. (1996). Concept analysis in nursing research: A critical appraisal. *Scholarly Inquiry for Nursing Practice: An International Journal*, 10, 253–277.

Rycroft-Malone, J. (2004). The PARIHS framework – A framework for guiding the implementation of evidence-based practice. *Journal of Nursing Care Quality*, 19(4), 297–304.

Rycroft-Malone, J. (2007). Theory and knowledge translation: Setting some co-ordinates? *Nursing Research*, 56(4S) S78–S85.

Rycroft-Malone, J., Kitson, A., Harvey, G., McCormack, B., Seers, K., Titchen, A., and Estabrooks, C.A. (2002). Ingredients for change: Revisiting a conceptual framework. *Quality and Safety in Health Care*, 11, 174–180.

Rycroft-Malone, J., Harvey, G., Seers, K., Kitson, A., McCormack, B., and Titchen, A. (2004a). An exploration of the factors that influence the implementation of evidence into practice. *Journal of Clinical Nursing*, 13, 913–924.

Rycroft-Malone, J., Seers, K., Titchen, A., Harvey, G., Kitson, A., and McCormack, B. (2004b). What counts as evidence in evidence-based practice. *Journal of Advanced Nursing*, 47(1), 81–90.

Rycroft-Malone, J., Fontenla, M., Seers, K., and Bick, D. (2009). Protocol-based care: The standardisation of decision making. *Journal of clinical Nursing*, 18, 1488–1498.

Sharp, N., Pineros, S.L., Hsu, C., Starks, H., and Sales, A. (2004). A qualitative study to identify barriers and facilitators to the implementation of pilot intervention in the Veterans Health Administration Northwest Network. *Worldviews on Evidence-Based Nursing*, 1(4), 129–139.

Sudsawad, P. (2007). *Knowledge Translation. Introduction to Models, Strategies and Measures.* Austin, TX: Southwest Education Development Laboratory, The National Center for the Dissemination of Disability Research. Available at: http://www.ncddr.org/kt/products/ktintro/ktintro. pdf (last accessed 1 July 2009).

Wallin, L., Estabrooks, C.A., Midodzi, W.K., and Cummings, G.G. (2006). Development and validation of a derived measure of research utilization by nurses. *Nursing Research*, 55(3), 149–160.

Wright, J., McCormack, B., Coffey, A., and McCarthy, G. (2007). Evaluating the context within which continence care is provided in rehabilitation units for older people. *International Journal of Older People Nursing*, 2(1), 9–19.

Chapter 6

Iowa model of evidence-based practice

Marita Titler

Key learning points

- The Iowa model of evidence-based practice (EBP) is a practice mode with the primary purpose of guiding practitioners (including physicians, nurses, allied health) in the use of evidence to improve healthcare outcomes.
- The model is based on planned action process, and incorporates conduct of research, use of research evidence, and other types of evidence.
- Assumptions underpinning the model are (a) working as a team is an important part of the applying evidence in practice, (b) evaluation is an essential part of the EBP process, and (c) EBP is a process not an event.

Overview and purpose

The Iowa model of evidence-based practice (EBP) is a *practice* model with the primary purpose of guiding clinicians (physicians, nurses, allied health care) in the use of evidence to improve health care outcomes (see Fig. 6.1). It incorporates conduct of research, use of research evidence, and other types of evidence such as case reports and expert opinion (Titler, 2009; Titler *et al.*, 2001). This process model has been widely disseminated and adopted in academic and

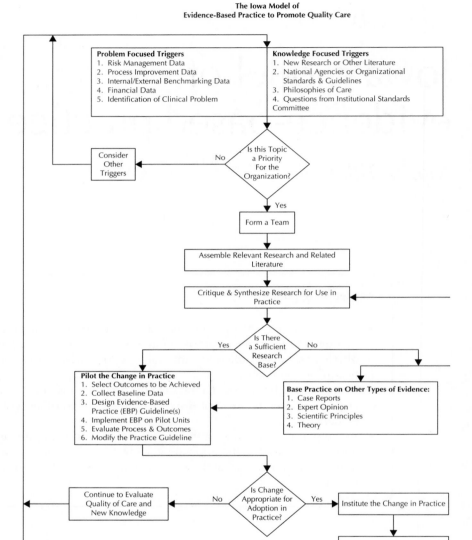

Figure 6.1 The Iowa model of evidence-based practice to promote quality care (adapted from Titler *et al.*, 2001)

clinical settings (Titler *et al.*, 2001). Since the original publication in 1994 (Titler *et al.*, 1994a), the authors have received over 1200 requests to use the model for publications, presentations, grant proposals, graduate and undergraduate courses, clinical research, and

EBP programs. It has been cited 95 times in nursing journal articles (Social Science Citation Index, June 25, 2008).

In this model, knowledge- and problem-focused "trigger(s)" lead staff members to question current health care practices and whether patient care can be improved through the use of research findings. If through the process of literature review and critique of studies, it is found that there is not a sufficient number of scientifically sound studies to use as a base for practice, consideration is given to conducting a study. Clinicians collaborate with scientists in nursing and other disciplines to conduct clinical research that addresses practice problems encountered in the care of patients. Findings from such studies are then combined with findings from existing scientific knowledge to develop and implement these practices. If there is insufficient research to guide practice, and/or conducting a study is not feasible, other types of evidence (e.g., case reports, expert opinion, scientific principles, theory) are used and/or combined with available research evidence to guide practice. Priority is given to projects in which a high proportion of practice is guided by research evidence. Practice guidelines usually reflect research and nonresearch evidence and therefore are called EBP guidelines.

An EBP guideline or detailed EBP standard is developed from the available evidence. The recommended practices, based on the relevant evidence, are compared to current practice, and a decision is made about the necessity for a practice change. If a practice change is warranted, changes are implemented using a process of planned change. The practice is first implemented with a small group of patients, and an evaluation is carried out. The EBP is then refined based on evaluation data, and the change is implemented with additional patient populations for which it is appropriate. Patient/family, staff, and fiscal outcomes are monitored. Organizational and administrative supports are important factors for success in using evidence in care delivery.

Assumptions implicit in the model include (a) working as a group/team is an important part of applying evidence in practice; (b) evaluation is essential part of the process of EBP; and (c) EBP is a process, not an event, that requires multiple steps to align clinician behavior and system support for delivery of evidence-based health care. Authors of the Iowa model adopted the definition of EBP as the conscientious and judicious use of current best evidence to guide health care decisions (Sackett *et al.*, 1996). Levels of evidence range from randomized clinical trials to case reports and expert opinion. Additional assumptions include that the model is applicable for various health care disciplines, not just nurses, and that improvement in processes and outcomes of health care are often interdisciplinary in nature, such as improving acute pain management of older adults.

Development of the model

The first version of the Iowa model (often called the 1994 version) was a culmination of the leadership of the Research Committee at the University of Iowa Hospitals and Clinics (UIHC) (Cullen *et al.*, 2005; Titler *et al.*, 1994b). This acute care academic medical center had been facilitating application of evidence in practice since 1986, under what was commonly referred to as research utilization. The Research Committee developed the original Iowa model flow diagram to illustrate the process used for research utilization by staff nurses at UIHC. The original flow diagram and accompanying narrative were published in Nursing Research (Titler *et al.*, 1994b) and subsequent to the publication, we received multiple requests for use of the model. In development of this process model, we sought feedback from our staff nurses; experts in research utilization such as Linda Cronenwett, and other nurse leaders. In 1998, the original model was revised and updated to be more in line with the current quality improvement and EBP literature, and was published in 2001 (Titler *et al.*, 2001). The model has been in place for over 20 years at UIHC.

The model was developed and applied in the context of acute care nursing practice. It was adopted as the model for quality improvement for all disciplines at UIHC and was discussed with regulatory agencies such as Joint Commission on Accreditation of Healthcare Organizations when they visited. The majority of requests for use of the model have come from hospitals ($n = 873$) and Colleges of Nursing ($n = 337$), but long-term care, public health agencies, and ambulatory settings have also requested use of the model ($n = 18$).

Theoretical underpinnings of the model come from quality and performance improvement, and organization and systems literature. For example, the decision point regarding "is this topic a priority for the organization" illustrates the importance of organizational support for implementing EBP. Similarly, the evaluation component, dissemination of evaluative findings, and the feedback loops illustrate the theoretical underpinnings of quality and performance improvement in the model. The model differentiates between conduct of research and the process of EBP, a type of quality improvement to improve patient outcomes.

The original and revised models were empirically developed using a deductive approach of multiple and repeated processes used by staff nurses to integrate evidence into practice. The model is subsequently used as a guide for clinicians regarding the process of improving care through the application of evidence in practice for various topics such as improvement in pain management, assessing return of bowel motility following abdominal surgery in adults, and transitioning care of pediatric patients from the critical care unit to the general ward. Multiple publications from staff at the University of Iowa illustrate the application of the model and include evaluative data regarding the impact of changes in practice (Bowman *et al.*, 2005; Cullen *et al.*, 1999; Gordon *et al.*, 2008; Hanrahan and Lofgren, 2004; Madsen *et al.*, 2005; Stebral *et al.*, 2006; Van Waning *et al.*, 2005). The model has also been used by others in their publications (Gawlinski and Rutledge, 2008; Kresse *et al.*, 2007 Ong *et al.*, 2009; Parker *et al.*, 2009; Witzke *et al.*, 2008) and we have processed 40 requests to include the Iowa model in review of EBP models.

Intended users

The intended audience for the Iowa model is practitioners. It addresses both the individual and organizational perspective of EBP because multifaceted active implementation strategies are needed to promote use of research evidence in clinical and administrative decision making (Squires *et al.*, 2007; Titler, 2008). It is appropriate for teams and organizations. An individual practitioner in isolation of others would have difficulty using this model because it promotes use of teams, garnering organizational support (e.g., selecting a topic of importance to the setting), changes in systems (e.g., documentation systems), and education and change of individual practice behaviors. Although originally designed for practice, the model has been adopted by some academic settings and used to integrate EBP content into the curricula for graduate and undergraduate courses. For example, we have processed 255 requests for use of the model in teaching, and 200 requests for use of the model in student papers. Authors of the model have presented multiple faculty workshops using the Iowa model, and consulted on curricular revisions to integrate EBP content.

The Iowa model is also used as the framework for the *Advanced Practice Institute: Promoting Adoption of Evidence-Based Practice*, a 3-day train-the-trainer program for EBP that began as an innovative program at the University of Iowa Hospitals and Clinics under the direction of Titler. The purpose of the Advanced Practice Institute is to educate nursing leaders to guide colleagues and staff in the integration of evidence-based knowledge into practice. The Institute has the following goals: (a) to promote advanced skills of nursing leaders in use of EBP models; (b) to develop leadership skills for facilitating completion of clinically relevant EBP projects; and (c) to foster networks for creative thinking and issue resolution in the EBP process. Over 25 training programs have been provided from 2002 through 2009 with attendees representing numerous states in the USA. The Iowa model is used as the guiding framework for the EBP Staff Nurse Internship Program held every 2 years at UIHC. This program guides a small cohort of staff nurses (six to eight per group) in improving care for a specified topic, and selects attendees from a competitive application process. Evaluation by participants demonstrated the positive impact of this program on knowledge and skills in applying evidence to improve patient outcomes. Evaluation data and details about this program are available elsewhere (Cullen and Titler, 2004).

Hypothesis generation

Although the Iowa model is a practice model rather than a research model, it has generated research hypotheses and been used in 19 grant proposals. Some of these proposals were seeking funds for education of clinicians in EBP, while others were large center grant proposals. For example, The Iowa model was central to the 15 years of NIH funding and work of the Research Translation and Dissemination Core of the Gerontological Nursing Intervention Research Center (PI Tripp-Reimer, P30 NR003979). The model was used as a guiding framework for a funded study by the Center for Disease Control regarding prevention and treatment of MRSA in Iowa (PI Herwaldt grant no. RFA CD-07-005). The model has also been used to guide assessment of knowledge, skills, and attitudes regarding research and EBP with subsequent educational programming for staff to improve use of evidence in practice (Witzke *et al.*, 2008).

The model has been tested and evaluated in acute care settings through numerous EBP projects on various topics such as assessing return of bowel sounds following abdominal surgery in adults, preventing aspiration with enteral feedings in adult critically ill patients (Bowman *et al.*, 2005), family pet visitation, family transition from PICU to the pediatric floor, suicide risk assessment, sedation management in mechanically ventilated patients, as well as other topics (Hanrahan and Lofgren, 2004; Ong *et al.*, 2009; Parker *et al.*, 2009; Witzke *et al.*, 2008). These case examples improved care with the application of evidence in practice, guided by the Iowa model. Another example, is use of the model at the McGill University Health Center in Montreal Canada first for addressing Basic Cardiac Life Certification, and now for other changes in practice (Covell, 2006). The model has also been evaluated by developers through the application in two programs designed for clinicians – the Staff Nurse Internship for EBP, and the Advanced Practice Institute for EBP designed for clinical leaders. These programs are described in the previous section of this chapter.

Critique (strengths and weaknesses) of the Iowa model

The major strengths of the model are that it guides users through the process of applying evidence in practice in acute care settings. It is intuitive for practitioners and decision points in the model assist in driving the process forward (Bliss-Holtz, 2007). It addresses selecting EBP topics that are priorities for the organization, and guides the user through implementation and evaluation of implementing the changes on patient and staff outcomes. The model is broadly applicable for various health care disciplines including physicians, nurses, physical therapists, and allied health personnel. A major limitation of the model is the focus on using teams of clinicians to address EBP issues, rather than individual practitioners.

Barriers and facilitators to model implementation

Barriers to use of the model include the need for at least one individual or governance group (e.g., the Research Committee) to have primary responsibility for guiding users through the EBP process. This requires use of mentors who know the process and steps in the model. To facilitate use of the model, we offer educational programs, short courses, an annual EBP preconference, and consultations on model implementation. Other factors that facilitate use of the model include the interdisciplinary perspective that can be used with EBP implementation, and evaluation of the practice changes. A further strength of the model is the integration with quality improvement that begins with topic selection and continues with using both baseline and follow-up data to sustain the improvements in care delivery.

Future plans for model revisions

The plans for updating the model include interviewing attendees of the Advanced Practice Institute for EBP to garner feedback regarding their use and suggested revisions. A questionnaire is currently under development for those who have sought permission to use the model to gain their suggestions for model improvement. This information will be analyzed by the model developers to revise the model, with the revised model disseminated for further comment by the users.

Summary: How the model can be used/applied

- For the development of curricula for EBP training and education programs (including graduate and undergraduate courses).
- To guide the processes of improving practice and patient outcomes based on evidence.
- To guide the assessment of knowledge, skills, and attitudes regarding research and EBP.
- It is appropriate for the use by teams and organizations.

References

Bliss-Holtz, J. (2007). Evidence-based practice: A primer for action. *Issues in Comprehensive Pediatric Nursing*, 30(4), 165.

Bowman, A., Greiner, J., Doerschug, K., Little, S., Bombei, C., and Comried, L. (2005). Implementation of an evidence-based feeding protocol and aspiration risk reduction algorithm. *Critical Care Nursing Quarterly*, 28(4), 324–333.

Covell, C. (2006). BCLS certification of the nursing staff: An evidence-based approach. Journal of Nursing *Care Quality*, 21(1), 63.

Cullen, L. and Titler, M.G. (2004). Promoting evidence-based practice: An internship for staff nurses. *Worldviews on Evidence-Based Practice*, 1(4), 215–223.

Cullen, L., Titler, M.G., and Drahozal, R. (1999). Family and pet visitation in the critical care unit. *Critical Care Nurse*, 19(3), 84.

Cullen, L., Greiner, J., Greiner, J., Comried, L., and Bombei, C. (2005). Excellence in evidence-based practice: An organizational and MICU exemplar. *Critical Care Nursing Clinics of North America*, 17(2), 127–142.

Gawlinski, A. and Rutledge, D.N. (2008). Selecting a model for evidence-based practice changes: A practical approach. *AACN Advanced Critical Care*, 19(3), 291–300.

Gordon, M., Bartruff, L., Gordon, S., Lofgren, M., and Widness, J. (2008). How fast is too fast? a practice change in umbilical arterial catheter blood sampling using the Iowa model for evidence-based practice. *Advances in Neonatal Care*, 8(4), 198.

Hanrahan, K. and Lofgren, M. (2004). Evidence-based practice: Examining the risk of toys in the microenvironment of infants in the neonatal intensive care unit. *Advances in Neonatal Care*, 4(4), 184–201, quiz 202.

Kresse, M., Kuklinski, M., and Cacchione, J. (2007). An evidence-based template for implementation of multidisciplinary evidence-based practices in a tertiary hospital setting. *American Journal of Medical Quality*, 22(3), 148.

Madsen, D., Sebolt, T., Cullen, L., Folkedahl, B., Mueller, T., Richardson, C., *et al.* (2005). Listening to bowel sounds: An evidence-based practice project. *American Journal of Nursing*, 105(12), 40-9, quiz 49–50.

Ong, J., Miller, P., Appleby, R., Allegretto, R., and Gawlinski, A. (2009). Effect of a preoperative instructional digital video disc on patient knowledge and preparedness for engaging in postoperative care activities. *Nursing Clinics of North America*, 44(1), 103.

Parker, G., McEver, M., Fanning, L., Siefke, A., and Dobbs, N., (2009). Do shoes matter? A story of shoes in the neonatal intensive care unit. *Journal of Nursing Administration*, 39(1), 1–3.

Reavy, K. and Tavernier, S. (2008). Nurses reclaiming ownership of their practice: Implementation of an evidence-based practice model and process. *The Journal of Continuing Education in Nursing*, 39(4), 166.

Sackett, D., Rosenberg, W., Gray, J., Haynes, R., and Richardson, W. (1996). Evidence based medicine: What it is and what it isn't. *British Medical Journal*, 312, 71–72.

Stebral, L.L., Steelman, V., and Pottinger, J. (2006). Double gloving for surgical procedures: An evidence-based practice project. *Perioperative Nursing Clinics*, 1(3), 251–260.

Squires, J.E., Moralejo, D., and LeFort, S.M. (2007). Exploring the role of organizational policies and procedures in promoting research utilization in registered nurses. *Implementation Science*, 2, 17.

Titler, M.G. (2008). The evidence for evidence-based practice implementation. In: Hughes, R (ed.). *Patient Safety & Quality - An Evidence-Based Handbook for Nurses*, 1st ed. Rockville, MD: Agency for Healthcare Research and Quality (http://www.ahrq.gov/qual/nurseshdbk/).

Titler, M.G. (2009). Developing an evidence-based practice. In: LoBiondo-Wood, G. and Haber, J. (eds). *Nursing Research: Methods and Critical Appraisal for Evidence-Based Practice*,. 7th ed. St. Louis, MO: Mosby, Inc.

Titler, M.G., Kleiber, C., Steelman, V., Goode, C., Rakel, B., Barry-Walker, J., *et al.* (1994a). Infusing research into practice to promote quality care. *Nursing Research*, 43(5), 307–313.

Titler, M.G., Moss, L., Greiner, J., Alpen, M., Jones, G., Olson, K., *et al.* (1994b). Research utilization in critical care: An exemplar. *AACN Clinical Issues*, 5(2), 124–132.

Titler, M.G., Kleiber, C., Steelman, V.J., Rakel, B.A., Budreau, G., Buckwalter, K.C., *et al.* (2001). The Iowa Model of evidence-based practice to promote quality care. *Critical Care Nursing Clinics of North America*,13(4), 497–509.

Van Waning, N., Kleiber, C., and Freyenberger, B. (2005). Development and implementation of a protocol for transfers out of the pediatric intensive care unit. *Critical Care Nurse*, 25(3), 50–55.

Witzke, A., Bucher, L., Collins, M., Essex, M., Prata, J., Thomas, T., *et al.* (2008). Research needs assessment: Nurses' knowledge, attitudes, and practices related to research. *Journal for Nurses in Staff Development*. 24(1), 12–18, quiz 19.

Chapter 7

Dissemination and use of research evidence for policy and practice

A framework for developing, implementing, and evaluating strategies

Maureen Dobbins

Key learning points

- The dissemination and use of research evidence for policy and practice model was developed to provide a guiding map to individuals and organizations in the health care field to assist them in achieving evidence-informed decision making.
- On the basis of the Diffusion of Innovations Theory, a synthesis of literature on organizational behavior, culture, and decision making from the management field, as well as studies published in the health literature on research dissemination, research utilization, and evidence-based practice (EBP).
- The model was designed to be used by a variety of users, from direct service delivery to provincial and federal policy settings.
- The model has been used by other researchers to develop and evaluate knowledge translation and exchange (KTE) strategies, as well as those in the practice setting to develop strategies within their organizations to facilitate evidence-informed decision

making. Modifications to the model have occurred based on user feedback.
- Assessment of these factors at the individual and organizational level is instrumental in assessing organizational readiness for evidence-informed decision making, as well as in identifying and modifying the KTE strategies to be implemented.

Introduction

Worldwide there is substantial political and societal pressure to demonstrate the integration of the best available research evidence along with local contextual factors, so as to provide the most effective health services. In doing so, it is assumed that optimal patient and population health outcomes will be realized (Lavis *et al.*, 2003). Evidence-informed decision making is the integration of research evidence into policy and program decision making (Lomas *et al.*, 2005), and strategies to promote it are known as knowledge translation and exchange (KTE). While definitive answers of how best to achieve evidence-informed decision making remain elusive, it is well known that the decision-making process is complex and that multiple forms of knowledge impact both the process as well as the decision. Factors known to contribute to decision making include past experiences, beliefs, values, skills, resources, legislation, protocols, patient preferences, societal norms, and research results (Estabrooks, 1998; Haynes, 2001; Kouri, 1997; Sibbald and Roland, 1997). The intent of evidence-informed decision making is to suggest that policy and program decisions be determined by integrating the best available research evidence alongside other forms of evidence in the decision-making process.

Barriers to evidence-informed decision making include: lack of time; limited access to research evidence; limited capacity to appraise and translate research evidence; and resistance to change (Ciliska *et al.*, 1999; Davis *et al.*, 1992a; Hunt, 1996; Pettengill *et al.*, 1994; Raudonis and Griffith, 1991; Shaperman, 1995; Stolk and Mayo, 1995). Currently, the evidence tells us that passive KTE strategies involving the pushing of evidence out to users or one-way dissemination, when used alone are relatively ineffective (Dobbins *et al.*, 2005b; Grol and Grimshaw, 2003). However, strategies that facilitate interaction and face-to-face contact show promising results (Davis *et al.*, 1992b; Dobbins *et al.*, 2005b; Lavis *et al.*, 2005; Lomas *et al.*, 1991; Oxman *et al.*, 1995), and decision maker involvement in the research process results in greater use of research uptake (Canadian Health Services Research Foundation, 1999; Cargo and Mercer, 2008; Kothari *et al.*, 2005).

Purpose of the framework

To date, many KTE models and frameworks have been developed in an attempt to explain the process(es) of evidence-informed decision making among various health care professionals and health care settings. The models and frameworks differ by their philosophical underpinnings, the literature used to develop them, and their suggested uses. This chapter focuses on one framework initially published in 2002 (Dobbins *et al.*, 2002) and further refined in 2005 (Dobbins *et al.*, 2005a) – *Dissemination and use of research evidence for policy and practice: A framework for developing, implementing, and evaluating strategies.*

According to definitions on Wikipedia, a conceptual framework is used in research to outline possible courses of action or to present a preferred and reliable approach to an idea or thought (http://en.wikipedia.org/wiki/Framework), and a model is a pattern, plan, representation (especially in miniature), or description designed to show the main object or workings of an object, system, or concept (http://en.wikipedia.org/wiki/Models). Based on these descriptions what is described in this chapter is a model of the process by which health care decision makers and organizations engage in evidence-informed decision making. The intent of the model is not to suggest testable hypotheses as would be expected in a framework, but rather to depict a process as well as the many convening factors involved in the process. It was also the authors' intent in developing this model that the process and suggested associations between factors would be explored in future research. At the time this model was first conceptualized (1997), there were limited examples of KTE models and frameworks that integrated knowledge from a multidisciplinary perspective (e.g., literature from health care, business, psychology, anthropology, etc.), to provide a comprehensive depiction of the evidence-informed decision-making process. The purpose for this model's development was to describe and depict the process of evidence-informed decision making that would be applicable for both health policy and clinical decision making.

Model development

One of the basic assumptions underlying this model is that the use of the best available evidence for health policy and practice decisions will result in the provision of health services that are more effective and thus yield better patient outcomes, than decisions made in the absence of this evidence. Another key assumption concerns the evidence itself. While it is recognized in this model that evidence stems from multiple sources, a key focus in this model is the integration of the best available research evidence (which is collected through scientifically rigorous means), within the decision-making process. The term scientifically rigorous refers to all forms of research paradigms including quantitative and qualitative research. The foundation of the model encourages the incorporation of all of the relevant research evidence required to address a specific policy and/or practice-based issue. This implies that for any given health problem relevant research evidence might include rigorously collected epidemiological data that identifies an issue; patient and/or societal perspectives on the importance of the issue as well as acceptability of the possible solutions to the problem; program evaluations and quantitative studies evaluating the effectiveness of interventions; and qualitative studies assessing patient and/or societal experiences and perceptions of the interventions as well as explanations for how and why interventions worked or did not work. The assumptions inherent in this model are that any or all of these sources of evidence, when integrated into the decision-making process will result in better informed decisions, leading to improved health care service delivery, and enhanced patient and population health. Finally, while the model depicts a process that suggests evidence-informed practice proceeds in a linear and sequential way from knowledge through to confirmation, in fact the process can start anywhere in the model, and individuals and organizations may not move through the process in a sequential way (Fig. 7.1).

Background

The initial version of the model (Dobbins *et al.*, 2002) was developed by synthesizing studies from several bodies of literature

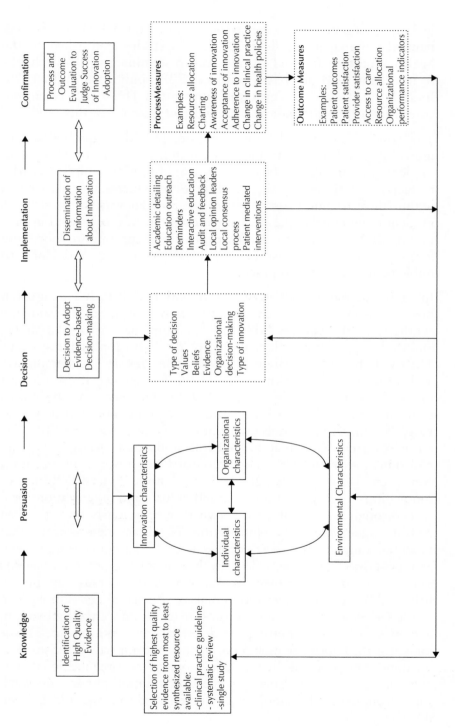

Figure 7.1 Framework for adopting an evidence-based innovation in an organization (adapted from Dobbins *et al.*, 2002)

including organizational behavior, culture, and decision making from the management field, as well as studies published in the health literature focused on research dissemination, research utilization, and evidence-based practice (EBP), published up to 1999. In addition, Roger's Diffusion of Innovation Theory provided and continues to provide the theoretical underpinnings of this model.

The primary intent of this model was to provide a guiding map to individuals and organizations in the health care field to assist them in identifying important factors they would need to address in order to facilitate EBP among their colleagues and themselves, as well as within their organization. Another major goal was to assist users in identifying appropriate dissemination strategies to be used in promoting EBP, as well as to identify realistic and appropriate short- and long-term outcome measures as a result of making a decision to implement evidence into practice.

In 1997 commonly used terms representing EBP included research dissemination and research utilization. As key messages from the synthesis of the various bodies of literature began to take shape, alongside a growing understanding of the Diffusion of Innovations Theory, it became apparent that the terms research dissemination and utilization mapped onto two of the five phases of diffusion of innovations described by Rogers (1995). Therefore, as the model evolved the five phases of the Diffusion of Innovations theory provided the underlying conceptualization of the process of EBP. The terms research dissemination, research utilization, decision making, and outcomes were then mapped onto the corresponding diffusion constructs (Dobbins *et al.*, 2002). For example, Rogers' Diffusion of Innovations Theory illustrates that individuals and organizations proceed through a series of actions (whether consciously or not) when considering adoption of an innovation. The theory demonstrates that potential adopters first must become aware of an innovation, known as the Knowledge phase. Adopters then assess the potential benefits and harms of the innovation, known as the Persuasion phase, followed by activities involved in making the actual decision, known as the Decision phase. If a decision is made to adopt the innovation, activities to facilitate putting the decision into action occur. This is known as the Implementation phase. Finally, the impact the decision has on important outcomes (e.g., patient outcomes, organizational outcomes), referred to by Rogers as the Confirmation phase is assessed. Input from the confirmation phase is then used to revisit the decision if needed.

We then mapped onto the Diffusion of Innovation Theory terms the relevant EBP terms (Dobbins *et al.*, 2002). For example, research dissemination (ways in which research knowledge is made available to potential users) was mapped onto the Knowledge phase. The term evidence-based decision making was mapped to the Decision phase, and research utilization was mapped to the Implementation phase. Finally we mapped the term outcomes to the Confirmation phase.

Through the integration of the Diffusion of Innovation terms with the EBP terms, a vision of the process began to take shape. Within each phase, additional details of the important factors were described further. For example, under the Knowledge phase, research dissemination strategies we listed in order of their known effectiveness among health professionals from most effective to least effective. Under the Persuasion phase, four types of characteristics that impact perceptions of the benefits or harms of the innovation we identified. Further still specific factors within each characteristic demonstrated in the literature to significantly impact perceptions we listed. Moving on to the Decision phase, factors associated with decision making identified in the literature as impacting on the decision-making process as well as the outcome of decisions we listed. At the Implementation phase, strategies to promote integration of the decision (e.g., adoption of research evidence into practice) into the organization we listed. Strategies listed in the model focused on concrete changes to the organization that had to be put in place in order to facilitate health professional behavior change. For example in adopting guidelines on the prevention of pressure ulcers, an organization might first have to reallocate resources such that appropriate mattresses can be purchased. Finally, in the Confirmation phase, relevant and realistic short- and long-term health and organizational outcomes are listed.

Since 1997 much has been learned about EBP and a great many papers have been published describing numerous aspects of the process. As a result some of our initial conceptualizations have changed, as well as the terms used to depict EBP. This has led to changes in the model as depicted in the book *Evidence-Based Nursing: A Guide to Clinical Practice* edited by DiCenso *et al.* (see also Dobbins *et al.*, 2005b). The most significant modifications to the model involved reconceptualizing the Knowledge, Implementation, and Confirmation phases. In this more recent version of the model, the Knowledge phase has been reconceptualized as the optimal process a health care professional or decision maker might take to identify the highest quality, most highly synthesized forms of evidence (e.g., practice guidelines). In other words, an organization faced with a policy or practice-based issue, would engage in activities to identify relevant evidence in the most synthesized form, of the highest methodological quality. With respect to the Implementation phase, this was reconceptualized as knowledge translation strategies that could be used by individuals and organizations to translate research evidence into practice. This included strategies for building capacity for evidence-informed decision making, promoting awareness of the necessary changes to practice, and facilitating an organizational culture for integrating evidence into practice (Dobbins *et al.*, 2005b). Finally, what were considered strategies for the Implementation phase in the initial version of the model (e.g., organizational changes required to bring about practice changes) became process outcomes under the confirmation phase (Dobbins *et al.*, 2005b). For example resource allocation, change in policies and procedures to reflect the evidence, and change in professional practice, in this revised model, now reflect measures of successful implementation and represent outcomes rather than strategies. When conceptualized in this way, the model is presented as a more useful tool for individuals and organizations to promote evidence-informed decision making in their organizations.

Finally, the latest revisions to the model reflect changes in terminology and interpretation of those terms in the knowledge translation field. For example, the term EBP has been replaced with the more encompassing term, evidence-informed decision making, and research dissemination has been expanded to represent KTE.

Intended audience

The expectation is that this model will be useful for a variety of users, from individuals to teams and organizations, from direct service delivery to provincial and federal policy settings. The model is most applicable for those in service provision and or policy settings, who are interested in facilitating evidence-informed decision making within their organization. It is less useful for a knowledge generating organization (e.g., research institutes), whose mandate is to promote the uptake of the knowledge they are generating to those in the service delivery or policy development.

More specifically, the intended audience could include a variety of individuals whose responsibility it is to facilitate evidence-informed decision making. This might include knowledge brokers, information specialists, advanced practice nurses, clinical nurse specialists, or project coordinators, and policy analysts. The titles vary from organization to organization and across the health professions. It may also include program managers who integrate the concepts of evidence-informed decision making into their everyday work. At an organizational level, organizations might use this model to assess various factors so as to identify where gaps exist, where additional capacity development is required, and where to focus their KTE efforts. Intended users are from the clinical setting in terms of service provision, as well as the policy setting, where health policies are developed.

Finally another key intended user of the model is undergraduate and graduate students in the health professions. At the undergraduate level, students in health professional degrees can use the model to understand the process of translating research evidence into practice, and can develop scenarios of how this would occur by working through the phases of the model. They may even use concepts from the model to develop a knowledge translation plan for research evidence during clinical placements. The model may also be helpful for graduate students in developing research proposals. The model may help these students to pinpoint specific phases of the evidence-informed decision-making process that they would like to study further, or develop KTE strategies that they might evaluate in various settings. Some students might even continue to modify the model based on their specific settings. In summary, the model is adaptable to many health care settings and for various health care professionals. Intended users range from individuals to teams to organizations, and come from the practice setting or the policy setting. The model is also intended for use by both undergraduate and graduate students in health-related programs.

Hypothesis generation

Hypotheses that we have generated and tested relate primarily to factors associated with the persuasion and decision phases of the model. For example, we hypothesized that characteristics of the organization (e.g., the value the organization places on using research evidence in decision making), would moderate the impact of KTE strategies; meaning those organizations that value research evidence to a greater extent will receive greater benefit from knowledge translation strategies. In a randomized controlled trial evaluating the impact of three knowledge translation strategies, we determined in fact that the value organizations place on research evidence in decision making does moderate the effect of the knowledge translation strategies (Dobbins *et al.*, 2009). We also hypothesized that knowledge translation strategies that address organizational barriers to evidence-informed decision making will be more effective than those that do not. While some evidence of this was observed in our randomized trial on a subsample of participants, we recommend that additional research is needed to more fully understand this phenomenon.

One hypothesis that has not been specifically tested, but has emerged from our model is that different knowledge translation strategies will be more or less effective in different settings based on the underlying organizational characteristics. For example, one knowledge translation strategy, may be effective in one setting but not another, because of differences in organizational factors. The results of our randomized controlled trial indicated that tailored messages (pushing out of synthesized key messages from research evidence to specific target audiences), had statistically significant positive effects *if* the organization highly valued the use of research evidence in decision making, but not when organizations did not value research evidence (Dobbins *et al.*, 2009). The inverse was observed for knowledge brokering (a trusted and respected expert in evidence-informed decision making worked one-on-one with decision makers to integrate research evidence into decision making). For organizations that did not value the use of research evidence the knowledge broker had a moderate positive effect. However, a knowledge broker had no impact on organizations that highly valued the use of research evidence (Dobbins *et al.*, 2009). We recommend that greater emphasis on assessing the factors identified in the persuasion phase of the model will lead to more appropriate knowledge translation strategies being identified and implemented, resulting in greater impact on evidence-informed decision making.

We have also hypothesized that many of the KTE strategies that currently exist would likely lead to significant and positive effects if implemented in the appropriate settings. Therefore, we suggest that assessment of the factors identified in the persuasion stage is an important component in identifying those KTE strategies that are most suitable and appropriate for that organization, and when implemented will yield that greatest benefit in terms of evidence-informed decision making.

Finally, from the decision phase of the model we hypothesized that the decision-making process is comprised of multiple components that impact the process including: who is participating in the decision, how the organization makes decisions, the importance of the decision to the mission of the organization; the magnitude of the decision in relation to resources and/or resource allocation; and perceptions of those involved in the decision in terms of what constitutes evidence. We explored this hypothesis through qualitative descriptive studies and have found this to be true (Dobbins *et al.*, 2007a). For example, depending on who is participating in the decision, what constitutes evidence for them and what implications the decision will have on resources, emerged as key themes among decision makers participating in our qualitative interviews (Dobbins *et al.*, 2007b).

Examples of framework's use

It is our perception that the model has been used frequently for multiple purposes, primarily in assisting individuals and organizations in developing a plan for promoting evidence-informed clinical practice. A search of Web of Science identified 16 citations in which either the 2002 (14 citations) or 2005 (2 citations) versions of the model were cited. We also have received multiple requests from graduate students as they use the model to frame their research projects.

Concepts from our model have been used in the development of other KTE models. In her model of Pathway's to evidence-informed policy, Bowen integrated concepts from our model into the policy-making process she describes. Specifically, she agreed with the factors we identified as affecting adoption of evidence at each step in the process of evidence-informed policy making, and also agreed with several of the factors we suggest impact on the decision-making process itself (Bowen and Zwi, 2005). Furthermore, in her depiction of the process of evidence-based decision making in Canada, components of our model are illustrated in recommendations for a Population and Public Health Evidence Centre suggested by Kiefer *et al.* (2005).

The model has also been cited in two systematic reviews evaluating KTE strategies including one in cancer control (Ellis *et al.*, 2005) and nurses' uncertainty in decision making (Cranely *et al.*, 2009), and one on organizing frameworks for KTE strategies (Mitton *et al.*, 2007). The model has also been cited in the background and or discussion section of published studies evaluating different factors associated with evidence-informed decision making as well as the effectiveness of knowledge translation strategies (Gagnon *et al.*, 2008; Genius, 2004; Gifford *et al.*, 2008; Jbilou *et al.*, 2007; Rappolt *et al.*, 2005; Zucker *et al.*, 2006).

One group of researchers and decision makers from Alberta, Canada, focused on developing appropriate, context-specific theories, and using theory to guide the evaluation and development of effective knowledge mobilization strategies, used our model as a basis for their work (Shaw, 2008). In modifying our model to better suit their needs in the context of children, youth, and families, Shaw *et al.* simplified the model to four components (knowledge mobilization activity, decision to adopt or reject, knowledge use, and outcomes), which are connected in a circular format (Shaw, 2008). The modified model is now guiding the identification of KTE strategies, their implementation into practice, as well as their evaluation (Shaw, 2008).

We are also aware of several researchers who have used the model in developing research proposals submitted to funding agencies in Ontario, Canada, and Australia. Some of the proposals that have received funding used the model to explore: the use of research evidence among those working in child welfare (Jack *et al.*, 2006), the effectiveness of a knowledge broker among those involved in policy development related to childhood obesity prevention (Waters *et al.*, 2006); and facilitating evidence-informed decision making among those working with women with substance use issues and their young children (Niccols *et al.*, 2008).

With respect to child welfare, a cross sectional study was conducted to explore decision maker's use of research evidence in decision making as well as characteristics associated with use. Similar results were found in the child welfare field (Jack, 2006), as have been reported previously for public health decision makers (Dobbins *et al.*, 2001).

A 5-year program of research, just underway among decision makers working with women with substance use issues and their young children, used our model to identify a series of consecutive studies related to KTE. Since no previous research has been done with this group of health professionals on evidence-informed decision making, our model was instrumental in depicting important constructs in the process for which specific research questions and studies were designed. For example the model assisted the researchers in designing an initial study to explore characteristics of the organizational, individual, and other factors identified in the persuasion phase as being associated with evidence-informed decision making, followed by a qualitative study to better understand the decision-making process and perceptions regarding what constitutes evidence in this field. The program of research will end with a study evaluating the feasibility of various KTE strategies among this population of health professionals.

Perceived strengths and weaknesses

Feedback received from users of the model has been both positive and negative. Positive comments have primarily been related to the ease of use of the model. For example, users have indicated that publications describing the model are easy for users to understand, interpret, and apply to their specific context. The model is easy to follow, and the phases and characteristics are described in sufficient detail that users understand what they need to assess and how to assess them. Users have also indicated that the model is useful for organizations in terms of identifying steps in the evidence-informed decision-making process and assisting them in identifying areas where the organization needs to develop capacity, as well as other areas where they have the needed skills and can leverage those skills for additional activities.

Feedback on weaknesses of the model include: it depicts too simplistic a view of the evidence-informed decision-making process; and that it appears too logical and rational. As the model is currently depicted, it appears as though decision making proceeds in a linear fashion, starting from the Knowledge stage of the model (becoming aware of research evidence) and ending at the confirmation stage (evaluation of outcomes resulting from implementing the KTE strategies). While this is not the intent of the model to suggest there is only one way to move through the process, the pictorial representation of the model does suggest this. Future work on the pictorial representation of the model needs to capture the complexities of the process, as well as the nonlinear process of evidence-informed decision making.

Another weakness of the model relates to context. While a number of organizational characteristics have been identified as important to the evidence-informed decision-making process, some have suggested that greater attention to context (organizational, environmental, and individual) needs to be built into the model. In addition, it has been suggested that the inclusion of concepts from Cognitive Behavioral Theory would contribute meaningfully to the model.

Barriers and facilitators to implementing the framework

Likely the most significant barrier to implementing our model is resources: both human and financial. The evidence-informed decision-making process as well as the implementation of KTE strategies to promote evidence-informed decision making, is not a short-term endeavor, and requires significant investment on the part of organizations and individuals. At the very least an organization must be willing to commit human resources to this activity, meaning one or more persons in the organization have as part of their job description, a responsibility to effect change in the organization that will result in evidence-informed decision making. This may require organizations to reallocate funding so as to finance new positions or free up personnel time from other responsibilities. This on its own may represent a significant barrier to implementing our model and engaging in the process of becoming an evidence-informed organization. However, in addition to the human resource issues, there are also significant costs associated with becoming an evidence-informed organization. For example, there may be costs incurred in providing professional development opportunities for individuals in the organization to develop skills and capacity for evidence-informed decision making. Organizations will also need to invest in a needs assessment, whether this is done in house or by an external consultant. It might also be that the needs assessment identifies processes in the organization that need to be developed or modified in order to promote and sustain evidence-informed decision making. All of these may result in significant costs to the organization that may represent substantial barriers to implementing our model and evidence-informed decision making.

In addition factors that may facilitate implementation of the model include a champion either internal or external to the organization, such as the chief executive officer or a professional association. We are currently aware of one such organization whose CEO has committed to a 10-year strategic plan to transform the organization into one which is evidence informed. Our model was useful in the very early days of this initiative, in terms of identifying the scope of work required to achieve this goal. Having the CEO as a champion of the process has been instrumental in ensuring the human and financial resources have been made available to position the organization to move forward with this objective. Another facilitator to implementation of the model is environmental or political factors. For example, the continuous quality improvement movement in health care is prompting organizations to become more efficient and effective. In doing so, there is the opportunity for organizations to achieve quality improvement by becoming evidence informed. This type of facilitator, which is largely out of control of health professionals and researchers, is likely to have the greatest impact on promoting evidence-informed decision making.

Future plans for framework modifications

Future plans for the model include continuing to explore the components of the model through both quantitative and qualitative research designs as well as continuing to test hypotheses stemming from the model. We expect over time as more knowledge is gained from these studies, as well as those of others, that modifications to the model will occur. We look forward to the model's evolution in the coming years (Table 7.1).

Summary: How the model can be used/applied

- The dissemination and use of research evidence model incorporates the stages of the Diffusion of Innovations to provide a guiding map to individuals and organizations to assist them in achieving evidence-informed practice. While there are many possible uses of the model, it could primarily be used to develop a step-by-step plan of implementing research evidence within an organization.
- The model should be useful for those charged with the responsibility in their organizations to integrate research evidence into practice as well as other researchers, graduate students, and research funders.

Table 7.1 Summary of model application

By whom	How	With whom	Types of projects
Knowledge brokers	• Face-to-face and electronic interaction • Individual and organizational needs assessments • Workshops	• Front line • Practitioners • Managers • Senior management • Health care organizations	• Capacity development in process of evidence-informed decision making • Working with specific individuals in an organization to incorporate research evidence into decision making
Information specialists	• Face-to-face interaction with practitioners	Frontline practitioners, managers, librarians	• To promote the use of research evidence in clinical practice • Skill development in question formulation
Clinical nurses specialists	• Identify barriers to guideline implementation • Engage stakeholders in process • Work to develop infrastructure and support to promote guideline implementation	Frontline nurses	• Promote uptake of best practice guidelines into organizational policy and practice
Advanced practice nurses	• Identify barriers to guideline implementation • Engage stakeholders in process • Work to develop infrastructure and support to promote guideline implementation	Frontline nurses	• Promote uptake of best practice guidelines into organizational policy and practice
Policy analysts	• Identify barriers to implementation evidence in policy • Engage stakeholders in process • Work to develop infrastructure and support to promote implementation of evidence in policy	Policy makers	• Promotion of use of evidence in the policy context • Development of skill in policy context for using research evidence in decision making

Table 7.1 (*Continued*)

By whom	How	With whom	Types of projects
Program managers	• Identify barriers to implementation evidence in policy • Engage stakeholders in process • Work to develop infrastructure and support to promote implementation of evidence in policy	Frontline staff, senior managers, relevant stakeholders	• Facilitate use of research evidence in program planning • Promote capacity among frontline staff and other program managers

- The Dissemination and Research Use model has been used in various ways including:
  - as a conceptual/theoretical framework for the development of research studies,
  - as the basis for modification of the model to suite different settings and health care professionals,
  - for developing and evaluating KTE intervention strategies.
- The components of the model have been used to develop a process for assessing individual and organizational barriers and facilitators for implementing research evidence into practice, developing KTE interventions, and in identifying relevant and appropriate individual and organizational level outcomes to be evaluated.
- The model offers the potential for hypothesis development, particularly in relation to intervention research.
- The model continues to be modified as new knowledge emerges from our own as well as other research in this field.

References

Bowen, S. and Zwi, A.B. (2005). Pathways to "evidence-informed" policy and practice: A framework for action. *PLoS Medicine*, 2, e166.

Canadian Health Services Research Foundation. (1999). Issues in linkage and exchange between researchers and decision-makers [on-line]. Available at: http://www.chsrf.ca/knowledge_transfer/pdf/linkage_e.pdf.

Cargo, M. and Mercer, S.L. (2008). The value and challenges of participatory research: Strengthening its practice. *Annual Review of Public Health*, 29, 325–350.

Ciliska, D., Hayward, S., Dobbins, M., Brunton, G., and Underwood, J. (1999). Transferring public-health nursing research to health-system planning: Assessing the relevance and accessibility of systematic reviews. *Canadian Journal of Nursing Research*, 31, 23–36.

Cranely, L., Doran, D., Tourangeau, A., Kushniruk, A., and Nagle, L. (2009). Nurses' uncertainty in decision making: A literature review. *Worldviews on Evidence-Based Nursing*, 6, 3–15.

Davis, D.A., Thomson, M.A., Oxman, A.D., and Haynes, R.B. (1992a). Evidence for the effectiveness of CME: A review of 50 randomized controlled trials. *Journal of the American Medical Association*, 268, 1111–1117.

Davis, D.A., Thomson, M.A., Oxman, A.D., and Haynes, R.B. (1992b). Evidence for the effectiveness of CME: A review of 50 randomized controlled trials. *JAMA*, 268, 1111–1117.

Dobbins, M., Cockerill, R., Barnsley, J., and Ciliska, D. (2001). Factors of the innovation, organization, environment, and individual that predict the influence five systematic reviews had on public health decisions. *International Journal of Technology Assessment in Health Care*, 17, 467–478.

Dobbins, M., Ciliska, D., Cockerill, R., Barnsley, J., and DiCenso, A. (2002). A framework for the dissemination and utilization of research for health-care policy and practice. *The Online Journal of Knowledge Synthesis for Nursing*, 9, 149–160.

Dobbins, M., Ciliska, D., Estabrooks, C., and Hayward, S. (2005a). Changing nursing practice in an organization. In A. DiCenso, G. Guyatt, and D. Ciliska (eds), *Evidence-Based Nursing: A Guide to Clinical Practice* (pp. 172–200). St. Louis, MO: Elsevier Mosby.

Dobbins, M., Davies, B., Danseco, E., Edwards, N., and Virani, T. (2005b). Changing nursing practice: Evaluating the usefulness of a best-practice guideline implementation toolkit. *Nursing Leadership*, 18, 34–48.

Dobbins, M., Rosenbaum, P., Plews, N., Law, M., and Fysh, A. (2007a). Information transfer: What do decision makers want and need from researchers? *Implementation Science*, 2, 20.

Dobbins, M., Jack, S., Thomas, H., and Kothari, A. (2007b). Public health decision-makers' informational needs and preferences for receiving research evidence. *Worldviews on Evidence-Based Nursing*, 4, 156–163.

Dobbins, M., Hanna, S., Ciliska, D., Thomas, H., Manske, S., Cameron, R., *et al.* (2009). A randomized controlled trial evaluating the impact of knowledge transfer and exchange strategies. *Implementation Science*, 4, 61.

Ellis, P., Robinson, P., Ciliska, D., Armour, T., Brouwers, M., O'Brien, M.A., *et al.* (2005). A systematic review of studies evaluating diffusion and dissemination of selected cancer control interventions. *Health Psychology*, 24, 488–500.

Estabrooks, C.A. (1998). Will evidence-based nursing practice make practice perfect? *Canadian Journal of Nursing Research*, 30, 15–36.

Gagnon, M.P., Legare, F., Fortin, J.P., Lamothe, L., Labrecque, M., and Duplantie, J. (2008). An integrated strategy of knowledge application for optimal e-health implementation: A multi-method study protocol. *BMC Medical Informatics and Decision Making*, 8, 17.

Genius, S.K. (2004). Exploring information context in the published literature of menopausal hormone therapy. *Libri*, 54, 199–210.

Gifford, W.A., Davies, B., Graham, I., Lefebre, N., Tourangeau, A., and Woodend, K. (2008). A mixed method pilot study with a cluster randomized controlled trial to evaluate the impact of a leadership intervention on guideline implementation in home care nursing. *Implementation Science*, 3, 51.

Grol, R. and Grimshaw, J. (2003). From best evidence to best practice: Effective implementation of change in patients' care. *Lancet*, 362, 1225–1230.

Haynes, R.B. (2001). Of studies, syntheses, synopses, and systems: The "4S" evolution of services for finding current best evidence. *Evidence Based Medicine*, 6, 36–38.

Hunt, J.M. (1996). Barriers to research utilization. *Journal of Advanced Nursing*, 23, 423–425.

Jack, S.M. (2006). Utility of qualitative research findings in evidence-based public health practice. *Public Health Nursing*, 23, 277–283.

Jack, S.M., Dudding, P., Dobbins, M., Tonmyr, L., and Kennedy, N. (2006). The Uptake and Utilization of Research Evidence by Child Welfare Policy Makers. The Provincial Centre of Excellence for Child and Youth at CHEO (unpublished work).

Jbilou, J., Amara, N., and Landry, R. (2007). Research based decision making in Canadian health organizations: A behvioural approach. *Journal of Medical Systems*, 31, 185–196.

Kiefer, L., Frank, J., Di Ruggiero, E., Dobbins, M., Manuel, D., Gully, P.R., *et al.* (2005). Fostering evidence-based decision-making in Canada: Examining the need for a Canadian Population and Public Health Evidence Centre and Research Network. *Canadian Journal of Public Health*, 96, I-1-I-19.

Kothari, A., Birch, S., and Charles, C. (2005). "Interaction" and research utilisation in health policies and programs: Does it work? *Health Policy*, 71, 117–125.

Kouri, D. (1997). *Introductory Module: Introduction to Decision Theory and Practice* Saskatoon, Saskatchewan, Canada: HEALNet.

Lavis, J.N., Robertson, D., Woodside, J.M., McLeod, C.B., Abelson, J., and Knowledge Transfer Study Group. (2003). How can research organizations more effectively transfer research knowledge to decision makers? *Milbank Quarterly*, 81, 221–248.

Lavis, J., Davies, H., Oxman, A., Denis, J.L., Golden-Biddle, K., and Ferlie, E. (2005). Towards systematic reviews that inform health care management and policy-making. *Journal of Health Services Research & Policy*, 10, 35–48.

Lomas, J., Enkin, M.A., Anderson, G.A., Hannah, W.J., and Singer, J. (1991). Opinion leaders vs audit and feedback to implement practice guidelines: Delivery after previous cesarean section. *JAMA*, 265, 2202–2207.

Lomas, J., Culyer, T., McCutcheon, C., McAuley, L., and Law, S. (2005). *Conceptualizing and Combining Evidence for Health System Guidance: Final Report*. Ottawa, ON: Canadian Health Services Research Foundation.

Mitton, C., Adair, C.E., McKenzie, E., Patten, S.B., and Waye Perry, B. (2007). Knowledge transfer and exchange: Review and synthesis of the literature. *Milbank Quarterly*, 85, 729–768.

Niccols, A., Dobbins, M., Sword, W., Henderson, J., Smith, P., Thabane, L., *et al.* (2008). Optimizing the Health of Women with Substance Use Issues and their Children. Canadian Institutes for Health Research.

Oxman, A.D., Thomson, M.A., Davis, D.A., and Hayes, J.E. (1995). No magic bullets: A systematic review of 102 trials of interventions to improve professional practice. *Canadian Medical Association Journal*, 153, 1423–1431.

Pettengill, M.M., Gillies, D.A., and Clark, C.C. (1994). Factors encouraging and discouraging the use of nursing research findings. *Journal of Nursing Scholarship*, 26, 143–147.

Rappolt, S., Pearce, K., McEwan, S., and Polatajko, H.J. (2005). Exploring organizational characteristics associated with practice changes following a mentored online educational module. *Journal of Continuing Education in the Health Professions*, 25, 116–124.

Raudonis, B.M. and Griffith, H. (1991). Model for integrating health services research and health care policy formation. *Nursing & Health Care*, 12, 32–36.

Rogers, E.M. (1995). *Diffusion of Innovations* (4th ed.) New York: The Free Press.

Shaperman, J. (1995). The role of knowledge utilization in adopting innovation from academic medical centers. *Hospital & Health Services Administration*, 40, 401–413.

Shaw, K.J.M. (2008). Knowledge Mobilization: Theory and Evaluation. In *Research Transfer Network of Alberta Conference*. Banff, Alberta.

Sibbald, B. and Roland, M. (1997). Getting research into practice. *Journal of Evaluation in Clinical Practice*, 3(1), 15–21.

Stolk, B.J. and Mayo, E. (1995). *Barriers to Research Utilization Perceived by Staff Public Health Nurses*. Ontario: University of Western Ontario.

Waters, E., Swinburn, B., Carter, R., Gold, L., Armstrong, R., Anderson, L., *et al.* (2006). A cluster randomized controlled trial of knowledge translation methods for obesity prevention. *National Medical Research Council of Australia* (unpublished work).

Zucker, D.R., Ruthazer, R., Schmid, C., Feuer, J., Fischer, P.A., Kieval, R.I., *et al.* (2006). Lessons learned combining N-of-1 trials to assess fibromyalgia therapies. *The Journal of Rheumatology*, 33, 2060–2077.

Chapter 8

ARCC (Advancing Research and Clinical practice through close Collaboration)

A model for system-wide implementation and sustainability of evidence-based practice

Bernadette Mazurek Melnyk and Ellen Fineout-Overholt

Key learning points

- The purpose of the Advancing Research and Clinical practice through close Collaboration (ARCC) model is to provide health care organizations and clinical settings with an organized conceptual framework that can guide system-wide implementation and sustainability of evidence-based practice (EBP) to achieve quality outcomes.
- The ARCC model is underpinned by Control Theory and Cognitive Behavioral Theory (CBT).
- The constructs in the model include culture and organizational readiness, the identification of facilitators and barriers, development and use of EBP mentors, and EBP implementation.
- Evidence includes research evidence, clinical expertise, and patient preference.

- Assessment and measurement tools are available for each stage of the EBP process represented in the model.
- The basic tenets that need to be in place for the ARCC model to be successful are: Inquiry is a daily part of the health care environment, quality outcomes are the overall goal, a process exists for the purpose of achieving the best outcomes, outcome and process data are transparent, clinicians are autonomous change agents, and health care is dynamic.

Although there are billions of dollars invested in research throughout the world to generate new knowledge and evidence to guide best practices, little of that evidence is actually implemented in clinical practice to improve health care quality and patient outcomes. Unfortunately, it takes an of average 17 years to translate evidence from research into clinical practice (Balas and Boren, 2000) due to multiple individual and system-wide barriers. As such, there is a tremendous need for conceptual models to guide health care organizations in implementing and sustaining evidence-based care throughout their entire systems by enhancing evidence-based practice (EBP) in individual clinicians and overcoming barriers to system-wide change.

Purpose of and assumptions in the ARCC model

The purpose of the Advancing Research and Clinical practice through close Collaboration (ARCC) model is to provide health care organizations and clinical settings with an organized conceptual framework that can guide system-wide implementation and sustainability of EBP to achieve quality outcomes. Since evidence-based clinicians are essential in cultivating an entire system culture that implements EBP as standard of care, the ARCC model encompasses key strategies for individual as well as organizational change to best practice.

Four important assumptions that are foundational to the ARCC model are:

(1) There are barriers and facilitators of EBP for individuals and within health care systems.
(2) Barriers to EBP must be removed or mitigated and facilitators put in place for both individuals and health care systems to implement EBP as standard of care.

(3) In order for clinicians to change their practices to be evidence-based, cognitive beliefs about the value of EBP and their confidence in their ability to implement it must be strengthened.

(4) A culture of EBP that includes EBP mentors (i.e., clinicians with advanced knowledge of EBP, mentorship, and individual as well as organizational change is necessary in order to advance and sustain individuals and health care systems' evidence-based care).

Background to the ARCC model

The ARCC model was originally conceptualized by Bernadette Melnyk in 1999 as part of a strategic planning initiative to unify research and clinical practice in order to advance EBP within an academic medical center for the ultimate purpose of improving health care quality and patient outcomes (Melnyk and Fineout-Overholt, 2002). Shortly following conceptualization of the ARCC model, advanced practice and point of care nurses in the medical center were surveyed about the barriers and facilitators of EBP. The results of this survey as well as Control Theory (Carver and Sheier, 1982, 1998) and Cognitive Behavioral Theory (CBT) (Beck *et al.*, 1979) guided the formulation of key constructs in the ARCC model. An important facilitator of EBP within the medical center identified by nurses who completed the survey was a mentor, which eventually became the key mechanism for implementing and sustaining EBP in both individual clinicians and health care systems in the ARCC model. Over the past decade, Melnyk and Fineout-Overholt have further developed the ARCC model through empirical testing of key relationships in the model and their extensive work with health care institutions to advance and sustain EBP.

Control Theory and Cognitive Behavioral Theory as a guide for the ARCC model

Control Theory (Carver and Scheier, 1982, 1998) contends that a discrepancy between a standard or goal (e.g., system-wide implementation of EBP) and a current state (e.g., the extent to which an organization is implementing EBP) should motivate behaviors in individuals to reach the standard or goal. However, in health care organizations, many barriers exist that inhibit clinicians from implementing EBP, including: (a) inadequate EBP knowledge and skills,

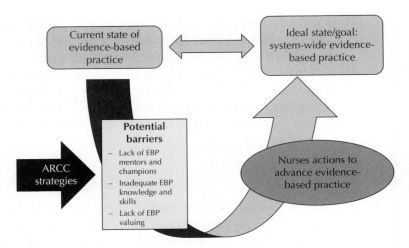

Figure 8.1 Control Theory as a conceptual guide for system-wide change to EBP in the ARCC model

(b) lack of administrative support, (c) lack of an EBP mentor, and (d) low beliefs that EBP improves patient care and outcomes) (Funk *et al.*, 1995; Hutchinson and Johnston, 2006; Melnyk and Fineout-Overholt, 2005). In the ARCC model, EBP mentors (i.e., clinicians who have in-depth knowledge and skills of EBP as well as individual and organizational change strategies [e.g., advanced practice clinicians – APCs]) are developed and placed within the health care system as a key strategy to mitigate or remove barriers commonly encountered by practicing clinicians in implementing EBP (see Fig. 8.1). As barriers lessen and the key facilitator of EBP (i.e., the mentor) is introduced, clinicians can implement EBP to improve quality of care and patient outcomes.

In the ARCC model, CBT is used to guide individual behavioral change toward EBP. CBT stresses the importance of individual, social, and environmental factors that influence cognition, learning, emotions, and behavior (Beck *et al.*, 1979; Lam, 2005). The basic premise of CBT is that an individual's behaviors and emotions are, in large part, determined by the way he or she thinks or his or her beliefs (i.e., the thinking–feeling–behaving triangle) (Melnyk and Moldenhauer, 2006). Based on CBT, a tenet of the ARCC model contends that when clinicians' beliefs about the value of EBP and their ability to implement it are strengthened, there will be greater implementation of evidence-based care. EBP mentors who work with point of care clinicians are critical to strengthening their beliefs about the value of EBP and their ability to implement it (see Fig. 8.2).

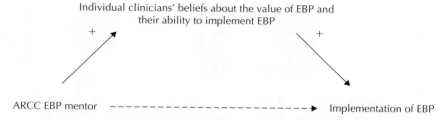

Figure 8.2 Cognitive Behavioral Theory as a conceptual guide for individual change to EBP in the ARCC model

Central constructs and relationships in the ARCC model

The first step in the ARCC model is an organizational assessment of culture and readiness for system-wide implementation of EBP (see Fig. 8.3). The culture of an organization can foster EBP or stymie it. If sufficient resources are not allocated to support the work of EBP, progress in advancing EBP throughout the organization will be slow. Administrators and point of care providers alike must adopt the EBP paradigm for system-wide implementation to be achieved and sustained. Assessment of organizational culture can be conducted with the use of the Organizational Culture and Readiness for System-wide Integration of Evidence-based Practice (OCRSIEP) scale (Fineout-Overholt and Melnyk, 2003). With the use of this 26-item Likert scale, a description of organizational characteristics, including strengths and opportunities for fostering EBP as well as barriers within a health care system are identified. Examples of items on the OCRSIEP scale include: (a) to what extent is EBP clearly described as central to the mission and philosophy of your institution, (b) to what extent do you believe that EBP is practiced in your organization, and (c) to what extent is the nursing staff with whom you work committed to EBP? The scale has established face and content validity, with internal consistency reliabilities consistently above 0.85 (Melnyk and Fineout-Overholt, 2011).

Once key facilitators and barriers to EBP are identified with the use of the OCRSIEP scale, a cadre of ARCC EBP mentors is developed within the health care system. EBP mentors are health care providers, typically APCs or baccalaureate prepared nurses where health systems do not have APCs, who work directly with point of care staff to implement EBP, including: (a) shifting from a traditional paradigm to an EBP paradigm, (b) conducting EBP implementation projects, and (c) integrating practice generated data to improve

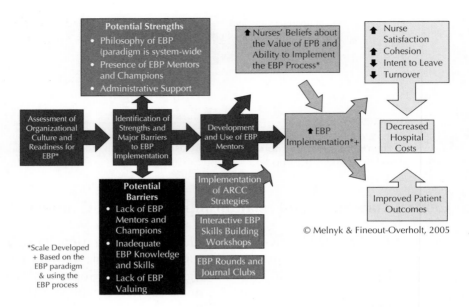

Figure 8.3 Melnyk and Fineout-Overholt's ARCC model (adapted from Melnyk and Fineout-Overholt © 2005)

health care quality as well as patient and/or system outcomes. EBP mentors also have knowledge and skills in individual behavior and organizational change strategies to facilitate changes in clinician behavior and spark sustainable changes in organizational culture, which require specific intervention strategies, time, and persistence. Intervention strategies include: (a) ongoing assessment of an organization's capacity to sustain an EBP culture, (b) building EBP knowledge and skills through conducting interactive group workshops and one-on-one mentoring, (c) stimulating, facilitating and educating nursing staff toward a culture of EBP, with a focus on overcoming barriers to best practice, (d) role modeling EBP, (e) conducting ARCC EBP-enhancing strategies, such as EBP rounds, journal clubs, web-pages, newsletters, and fellowship programs, (f) working with staff to generate internal evidence (i.e., practice-generated) through outcomes management and EBP implementation projects, (g) facilitating staff involvement in research to generate external evidence, (h) using evidence to foster best practice, and (i) collaborating with interdisciplinary professionals to advance and sustain EBP. These EBP mentors also have excellent strategic planning, implementation, and outcomes evaluation skills so that they can monitor the impact of their role and overcome barriers in moving the system to a culture of best practice (Melnyk, 2007). Mentorship with direct care staff on clinical units by ARCC EBP mentors is essential to strengthening clinicians' beliefs about the value EBP and their ability to implement it (Melnyk and Fineout-Overholt, 2002).

In the ARCC model, beliefs about the value of EBP and a clinician's ability to implement it foster EBP implementation using the EBP paradigm and subsequently improved outcomes. Clinicians' beliefs are measured with the EBP Beliefs (EBPB) scale (Melnyk and Fineout-Overholt, 2003). This is a 16-item Likert scale with responses that range from 1 (*strongly disagree*) to 5 (*strongly agree*). Examples of items on the EBPB scale include: (a) I am clear about the steps in EBP, (b) I am sure that I can implement EBP, and (c) I am sure that evidence-based guidelines can improve care. Item scores are summed to create a total EBP score, with higher scores indicating stronger EBP beliefs. The EBPB scale has established face, content, and construct validity, with internal consistency reliabilities consistently above 0.85 (Melnyk *et al.*, 2008). In the ARCC model, higher beliefs about EBP are expected to increase EBP implementation and, thereby, improve health care outcomes.

Evidence-based practice implementation in the ARCC model is defined as practicing based on the EBP paradigm. This paradigm uses the EBP process to improve outcomes. The process begins with asking clinical questions and incorporates research evidence and practice-based evidence in point of care decision making. However, simply engaging the process is not sufficient. The results of the first steps of the process (i.e., establishing valid and reliable research evidence) must be coupled with: (a) the expertise of the clinician to gather practice-based evidence (i.e., data from practice initiatives such as quality improvement [QI]), (b) gathering, interpreting, and acting on patient data as well as effectively using health care resources, and (c) determining what the patient and family values and prefers (see Fig. 8.4). This amalgamation leads to innovative decision making at the point of care with quality outcomes as the final product. While research evidence, practice evidence, and patient/client data as interpreted through expertise and patient preferences must always be present, the context of caring allows each patient–provider encounter to be individualized. Within an organization that fosters an EBP culture, this paradigm can thrive at the patient provider level as well as across the organization resulting in transformed health care.

Evidence-based practice implementation in the ARCC model is measured with the EBP Implementation (EBPI) scale, which is an 18-item Likert scale that measures the extent to which a clinician

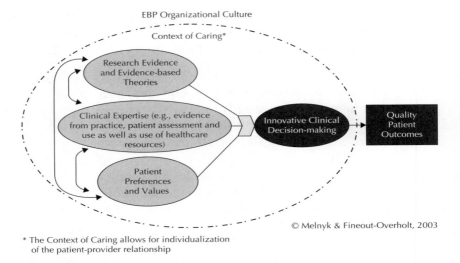

* The Context of Caring allows for individualization
  of the patient-provider relationship

Figure 8.4 Conceptual framework that underpins the EBP paradigm (adapted from Melnyk and Fineout-Overholt © 2003)

is implementing EBP. Clinicians respond to each of the items on the EBPI by answering how often in the last 8 weeks they have performed certain EBP tasks, such as: (a) generated a PICO question about my practice, (b) used evidence to change my clinical practice, (c) evaluated the outcomes of a practice change, and (d) shared the outcome data collected with colleagues. Item scores are summed for a total score, with higher scores indicating greater implementation of EBP. The EBPI has established face, content, and construct validity as well as internal consistency reliabilities above 0.85 (Melnyk *et al.*, 2008). In the ARCC model, it is contended that EBP implementation will improve health care outcomes through greater participation in evidence-based care. As well, EBP implementation is expected to be highly associated with higher nurse satisfaction, which will eventually lead to less turnover rates and health care expenditures.

Tenets of the ARCC model

There are some basic tenets that must be in place for the ARCC model to be successful:

(1) inquiry is a daily part of the health care environment;
(2) quality outcomes are the overall goal;

(3) process exists for the purpose of achieving the best outcomes;
(4) outcome and process data are transparent;
(5) clinicians are autonomous change agents;
(6) health care is dynamic.

As these tenets are evidenced in an organization, EBP can thrive. When there are barriers in the system that thwart the fulfillment of these tenets, EBP is less than successful as are health care outcomes. As the ARCC model has been refined, hypotheses that validate these tenets have been raised and tested.

Intended users

Intended users of the ARCC model include advanced practice nurses and transdisciplinary clinicians whose role it is to advance EBP in health care systems. In addition, directors of professional practice and research as well as chief executive and nursing officers in health care systems can use the model for strategic planning in creating system-wide implementation and sustainability of EBP. Nurse managers also can use the model to move the staff on their units to EBP implementation. The ARCC model also can be used by individual clinicians who are striving to understand what is necessary on an individual level to acquire EBP knowledge and skills as their standard practice paradigm. Lastly, there is a need for researchers to continue to test the role of the ARCC EBP mentor in improving clinicians' EBP beliefs and implementation as well as to gather additional supporting evidence for the various relationships in the model.

Hypotheses generated from the ARCC model

- There are positive relationships among EBP culture, clinicians' beliefs about EBP, and their implementation of EBP*.
- There is a positive relationship between clinicians' beliefs about EBP and their implementation of EBP*.
- There are positive relationships among clinicians' beliefs about EBP, implementation of EBP, and their role satisfaction*.
- Clinicians who practice in organizations with stronger EBP cultures versus those who practice in organizations with weaker EBP cultures will have stronger EBP beliefs and greater implementation of EBP.

- Clinicians who practice in organizations with stronger EBP cultures versus those who practice in organizations with weaker EBP cultures will report greater role satisfaction and less intent to leave.
- Health care systems that implement the ARCC model in which there is a cadre of EBP mentors will have stronger EBP cultures, greater implementation of EBP, higher nurse satisfaction, and less nurse turnover*.
- Health care systems in which clinicians report greater implementation of EBP versus those in which clinicians report lower implementation of EBP will have less turnover rates and better quality indicators.

The hypotheses designated with asterisks have been fully or partially supported through research, while future research is needed to test the others.

Research evidence to support the ARCC model

Research to support the relationships depicted in the ARCC model has been conducted and is ongoing. In one study (Melnyk *et al.*, 2004), a descriptive survey with a convenience sample of 160 nurses who were attending EBP conferences or workshops in four states located within the eastern region of the USA was conducted in order to: (a) describe nurses' knowledge, beliefs, skills, and needs regarding EBP, (b) determine whether relationships exist among these variables, and (c) describe major barriers and facilitators to EBP. Although participant beliefs about the benefit of EBP were high, knowledge of EBP was relatively low. Significant relationships were found between the extent to which the nurses' practice is evidence-based and: (a) nurses' knowledge of EBP, (b) nurses' beliefs about the benefits of EBP, (c) having an EBP mentor, and (d) using the Cochrane database of systematic reviews and the National Guidelines Clearinghouse. Findings from this study provided additional support for barriers and facilitators in the ARCC model as well as evidence to support the relationship between EBP beliefs and EBP implementation.

From this initial study, separate EBP beliefs and EBP implementation scales were developed in order to more fully study these constructs in the context of the ARCC model. Next, an instrumentation study was conducted to determine the psychometric properties of these EBP beliefs and the EBPI scales. A total of 394 nurses who attended continuing education workshops volunteered to complete the scales.

Data were analyzed to evaluate the validity and the reliability of both instruments. Principal components analyses indicated that each scale measured a unidimensional construct. Cronbach alphas for the two scales were above 0.90. Furthermore, findings indicated that the strength of nurses' EBP beliefs and EBP implementation increased as their educational level and responsibility in workplace roles increased. In addition, EBP beliefs and EBP implementation scores were highly correlated. Specifically, as EBP beliefs increased, EBP implementation increased.

In order to evaluate implementation of the ARCC model and determine the preliminary efficacy of having an ARCC mentor in a health care system on nurse outcomes, a randomized controlled pilot study was conducted with 47 nurses from three regions of a Visiting Nurse Service in downstate New York (USA). The regions were randomly assigned to either receive the ARCC intervention (i.e., having an EBP mentor) or an attention control intervention that focused on teaching the nurses in-depth physical assessment skills. The EBP mentor provided the nurses in the ARCC group with: (a) didactic content on EBP basics, (b) an EBP Toolkit, (c) environmental prompts (e.g., posters that encourage the nurses to use EBP), and (d) on-site and e-mail consultation about implementing an EBP project to improve patient outcomes. The ARCC EBP intervention program lasted 16 weeks, including a 4-week training period followed by the EBP mentor being on site with the nurses for 2 h one day a week for 12 weeks. Findings indicated that the ARCC group, compared to the attention control group had higher EBP beliefs, greater EBP implementation, and less nurse attrition/turnover. In addition, there was no significant difference between the ARCC and control groups on the outcome variable of nurses' productivity, indicating that nurse involvement in learning about how to integrate EBP into their daily practice along with implementing an EBP project during work time did not affect the number of home visits made by the nurses (Levin, pers. comm., 2006). Findings from this study support the positive outcomes of implementing the ARCC model in clinical practice.

Use and implementation of the ARCC model and implications for future research

The authors of the ARCC model have conducted national weeklong EBP mentorship immersion workshops that have prepared over 250 nurses and interdisciplinary clinicians across the nation and globe as ARCC EBP mentors. They have launched the nation's first 17-credit online EBP graduate certificate program that prepares expert EBP mentors through the Center for the Advancement of Evidence-based Practice at Arizona State University. Several individuals who have attended these workshops and certificate program have negotiated roles as EBP mentors within their health care organizations. Their roles range from point of care EBP mentors to directors of EBP who are responsible for creating a culture of EBP throughout their agencies. The ARCC initiatives that EBP mentors have used to promote and sustain implementation of EBP are as varied as the agencies from which they come, ranging from more traditional continuing education offerings to comedic videos about the role of EBP in addressing sacred cows. Not all EBP mentors who have put forth extensive efforts to advance EBP have experienced success reporting that the major barrier to their initiatives had been systems generated, which is another indication that an organizational culture of EBP is imperative for EBP to thrive.

In addition to individual EBP mentors, several hospitals throughout the USA have adopted the ARCC model in their efforts to implement and sustain EBP within their organizations. Organizational culture change and preparing of a critical mass of clinicians with at least beginning knowledge and skills in EBP are part of the preparation for establishing the ARCC model in an agency. Data collection is ongoing in these health care systems to determine the outcomes of implementing the ARCC model. Research also is currently underway to gather additional evidence to support the relationships in the ARCC model and establish outcomes of the ARCC EBP mentor within health care systems as the mentor role may very well be the key to sustainability of EBP in health care organizations (Melnyk, 2007).

Barriers and facilitators to implementing the ARCC model

When an organization considers adoption of the ARCC model, it is important that there is a commitment to changing the organizational paradigm and culture to EBP. However, it must be realized that cultural change is often slow and requires persistence. This may be perceived as a barrier to implementing the ARCC model.

When the investment is made by an organization to create a cadre of EBP mentors and build EBP knowledge and skills in their point of care staff, there needs to be a return on the investment that is demonstrated through outcomes evaluation. Another barrier could be evaluation of the impact of the ARCC model if an organization is not well versed in outcomes measurement.

Before adopting any EBP model, it is best for an agency to consider the investment required, particularly with the current economic climate, and how to capture the return on the investment. A caveat to keep in mind is that there may be a temptation to consider the venture required to adopt the ARCC model as an expense rather than an investment. However, implementation of the ARCC model promises long-term gains in quality outcomes as well as clinician satisfaction that must be considered when making decisions about which model(s) would provide the best return for the investment.

The most significant facilitator of the ARCC model is the EBP mentor. These uniquely prepared professionals drive the model's implementation and sustainability. Another facilitator is like-mindedness in terms of endorsing the EBP paradigm among administrators, leadership, and point of care providers. Having quality outcomes as the driver for decision making facilitates data transparency and fosters collaborative practice.

Critique (strengths and weaknesses) of the ARCC model

The ARCC model is intuitively welcomed by clinicians. Those who have experienced mentorship in other areas recognize the value of EBP mentors in sustaining health care improvement efforts. A strength of the ARCC model is its broad focus on systems and its accommodation of individual assimilation of the EBP paradigm. The active incorporation of clinician expertise is another strength of the ARCC model that allows any clinician, no matter what their professional tenure, to actively contribute to quality patient outcomes.

The ARCC model was designed to provide guidance to health care organizations and systems (e.g., tertiary care, primary care, long-term care, community and public health) as they systematically advance and sustain the EBP paradigm. The ARCC model also provides a context for generating research that can answer clinical questions for which there is insufficient valid and reliable evidence.

Limitations to the model include the need for further model testing and the conduct of further randomized controlled trials to establish the efficacy of the ARCC EBP mentor across various types of health care systems. However, given its beginning evidence and the established instruments to measure several constructs in the model, there is outstanding potential for transforming health care through the adoption of the ARCC model.

Summary: How the model can be used/applied

- To foster system-wide implementation and sustainability of EBP in health care institutions.
- To incorporate assessment data about a health care system's readiness for and culture of evidence-based practice (EBP) into strategic planning to integrate EBP into the fabric of the organization.
- To incorporate clinicians' EBP beliefs and implementation of EBP into strategies to enhance excellence in daily practice.
- To guide implementation strategies to strengthen clinicians' beliefs and implementation of EBP across the organization and at the point-of-care.
- To prepare advanced practice nurses and other clinicians to function as EBP mentors in a health care setting or system to sustain daily practice based on evidence.
- To generate research to further support the relationships in the ARCC model.

References

Balas, E.A. and Boren, S.A. (2000). Managing clinical knowledge for healthcare improvements. In: V. Schattauer (ed.), *Yearbook of Medical Informatics* (pp. 65–70). New York: Stuttgart.

Beck, A., Rush, A., Shaw, B., and Emery, G. (1979). *Cognitive Therapy of Depression*. New York: The Guilford Press.

Carver, C.S. and Scheier, M.F. (1982). Control theory: A useful conceptual framework for personality – Social, clinical, and health psychology. *Psychological Bulletin*, 92, 111–135.

Carver, C.S. and Scheier, M.F. (1998). *On the Self-Regulation of Behavior*. Cambridge, UK: Cambridge University Press.

Fineout-Overholt, E. and Melnyk, B.M. (2003). *The Organizational Culture and Readiness for System-wide Integration of Evidence-based Practice (OCRSIEP) Scale*. Rochester, New York: ARCC.

Funk, S. G., Tornquist, E. M., and Champagne, M. T. (1995). Barriers and facilitators of research utilization: An integrative review. *Nursing Clinics of North America*, 30, 395–407.

Hutchinson, A.M. and Johnston, L. (2006). Beyond the BARRIERS Scale: Commonly reported barriers to research use. *Journal of Nursing Administration*, 36(4), 189–199.

Lam, D. (2005). A brief overview of CBT techniques. In: S. Freeman and A. Freeman (eds), *Cognitive Behavior Therapy in Nursing Practice*. New York: Springer Publishing Company.

Melnyk, B.M. (2007). The evidence-based practice mentor: A promising strategy for implementing and sustaining EBP in healthcare systems [Editorial]. *Worldviews on Evidence-Based Nursing*, 4(3), 123–125.

Melnyk, B.M and Fineout-Overholt, E. (2002). Putting research into practice. *Reflections on Nursing Leadership*, 28(2), 22–25.

Melnyk, B.M. and Fineout-Overholt, E. (2003). *The Evidence-based Practice Beliefs Scale*. Rochester, New York: ARCC.

Melnyk, B.M. and Fineout-Overholt, E. (2005). *Evidence-Based Practice in Nursing and Healthcare. A Guide to Best Practice*. Philadelphia, PA: Lippincott, Williams & Wilkins.

Melnyk, B.M. and Moldenhauer, Z. (2006). *The KySS Guide to Child and Adolescent Mental Health Screening, Early Intervention and Health Promotion*. Cherry Hill, NJ: NAPNAP.

Melnyk, B.M., Fineout-Overholt, E., Feinstein, N., Li, H.S., Small, L., Wilcox, L., and Kraus, R. (2004). Nurses' perceived knowledge, beliefs, skills, and needs regarding evidence-based practice: Implications for accelerating the paradigm shift. *Worldviews on Evidence-based Nursing*, 1(3), 185–193.

Melnyk, B.M., Fineout-Overholt, E., and Mays, M. (2008). The evidence-based practice beliefs and implementation scales: Psychometric properties of two new instruments. *Worldviews on Evidence-Based Nursing*, 5(4), 208–216.

Melnyk, B.M. and Fineout-Overholt, E. (2011). *Evidence-Based Practice in Nursing and Healthcare. A Guide to Best Practice* (2nd edn). Philadelphia, PA: Lippincott, Williams & Wilkins.

Chapter 9

The Joanna Briggs Institute model of evidence-based health care as a framework for implementing evidence

Alan Pearson

Key learning points

- The Joanna Briggs Institute (JBI) model was developed in 2005 based on the work and underpinning methods and approach to evidence and evidence review within the JBI since over the preceding years.
- The JBI model describes the four major components of the evidence-based health care process as: health care evidence generation, evidence synthesis, evidence/knowledge transfer, and evidence utilization.
- JBI model acknowledges evidence derived from a wide range of research as legitimate evidence to inform practice.
- The three elements of the model concerned with evidence utilization (implementation), including: practice change; embedding

> evidence through system/organizational change; and evaluating the impact of the utilization of evidence on the health system.
> - The JBI tools provide an approach to implementing evidence-based criteria and a process of measuring outcomes in an identified area of practice.

Purpose and assumptions

This chapter examines *the Joanna Briggs Institute (JBI) model of evidence-based health care* (Pearson *et al.*, 2005) and the processes of implementing and embedding evidence in practice.

Evidence/knowledge translation in health care is particularly challenging to the evidence-based practice movement because it often requires investment at both the organizational and practitioner levels and the use of multiple strategies and interventions. Essentially, implementing evidence represents the age-old problem of health care: how to manage change.

There will never be an easy, one-size-fits-all solution to our ongoing problems associated with changing our practices and how we feel about change and the JBI model is essentially a framework for evidence-based health care that encourages the use of other models and frameworks.

Background to the JBI model's development

The JBI model was developed in 2005 based on the work and underpinning methods and approach to evidence and evidence review within the JBI over the preceding 9 years.

The JBI model

The JBI model describes the four major components of the evidence-based health care process as:

- Health care evidence generation.
- Evidence synthesis.
- Evidence/knowledge transfer.
- Evidence utilization.

Each of these components incorporate a number of essential elements; and the achievement of improved global health is seen as both the goal or endpoint of any or all of the model components and the "driving force" of evidence-based health care (Fig. 9.1).

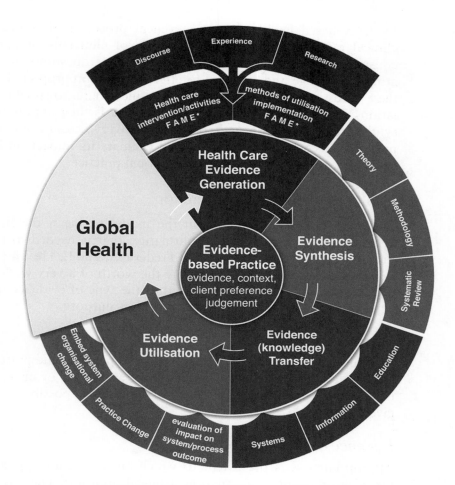

JBI Model of Evidence-Based Health Care

*FAME

Feasibility
Appropriateness
Meaningfulness
Effectiveness

Pearson A, Wiechula R, Court A and Lockwood C. 2005.
The JBI model of evidence-based healthcare
Int J Evid Based Healthc 3(8): 207-215.

Figure 9.1 Components of JBI model of evidence-based health care (adapted from Pearson *et al.*, 2005)

Evidence-based health care is a cyclical process that begins with clinical questions, concerns or interests of clinicians or patients/consumers, and then proceeds to address these questions by generating knowledge and evidence to effectively and appropriately meet these needs in ways that are feasible and meaningful to specific populations, cultures, and settings. This evidence is then appraised and synthesized and transferred to service delivery settings and health professionals who then utilize it and evaluate its impact on health outcomes, health systems, and professional practice.

Health care evidence generation

The term "evidence" is used in the model to mean the basis of belief; the substantiation or confirmation that is needed to believe that something is true (Miller and Fredericks, 2003). Health professionals seek evidence to substantiate the worth of a very wide range of activities and interventions and thus the type of evidence needed depends on the nature of the activity and its purpose.

Evidence of "feasibility"

Feasibility is the extent to which an activity is practical and practicable. Clinical feasibility is about whether or not an activity or intervention is physically, culturally, or financially practical or possible within a given context.

Evidence of "appropriateness"

Appropriateness is the extent to which an intervention or activity fits with or is apt in a situation. Clinical appropriateness is about how an activity or intervention relates to the context in which care is given.

Evidence of "meaningfulness"

Meaningfulness relates to the way in which an intervention or activity is understood by those who experienced or administer it. Meaningfulness arises out of the personal experience, opinions, values, thoughts, beliefs, and interpretations of patients, clients, or health professionals.

Evidence of "effectiveness"

Effectiveness is the extent to which an intervention, when used appropriately, achieves the intended effect. Clinical effectiveness is about the relationship between an intervention and clinical or health outcomes.

The Evidence Generation component of the model identifies opinion (discourse), experience, and research as legitimate means of evidence or knowledge generation. The means of generation are linked to the purpose of evidence generation in evidence-based health care, that is, to establish the feasibility, appropriateness, meaningfulness, or effectiveness of an intervention, activity, or phenomena in relation to both health care and to methods of using evidence and, thus, changing practices. Any indication that a practice is effective, appropriate, meaningful, or feasible; whether derived from experience or expertise or inference or deduction or the results of rigorous inquiry – is regarded as a form of evidence in the model. (The results of well-designed research studies grounded in any methodological position are, of course, seen to be more credible as evidence than anecdotes or personal opinion, however, when no research evidence exists, expert opinion is seen to represent the "best available" evidence.)

Evidence synthesis

The evaluation or analysis of research evidence and opinion on a specific topic to aid in decision making in health care consists of three elements in the model: theory, methodology, and the systematic review of evidence.

Although the science of evidence synthesis has developed most rapidly in relation to the meta-analysis of numerical data linked to theories of cause and effect, the further development of theoretical understandings and propositions of the nature of evidence and its role in health care delivery and the facilitation of improved global health is identified as an important element of this component of the model. Similarly, the increasing, ongoing interest and theoretical work on methods of synthesizing evidence from diverse sources is depicted as an element of evidence synthesis. The third element of evidence synthesis is the operationalization of methods of synthesis through the systematic review process. This element in the model is grounded in the view that evidence of feasibility, appropriateness, meaningfulness, effectiveness, and economics are legitimate foci for the systematic review process; and that diverse forms of evidence (from experience, opinion, and research that involves numerical and/or textual data) can be appraised, extracted, and synthesized (Pearson, 2004).

The systematic review and the synthesis of findings has its origins in quantitative psychology and the classical randomized controlled trial approach to clinical research in the health science fields. *The JBI model of evidence-based health care* adopts a pluralistic approach to the notion of evidence whereby the findings of qualitative research studies are regarded as rigorously generated evidence and other text derived from opinion, experience, and expertise is acknowledged as forms of evidence when the results of research are unavailable.

The core of evidence synthesis is the systematic review of the literature on a particular condition, intervention, or issue. The systematic review is essentially an analysis of all of the available literature (i.e., evidence) and a judgment of the effectiveness or otherwise of a practice, involving a series of complex steps.

Systematic reviews occupy the highest position in current hierarchies of evidence because they systematically search, identify, and summarize the available evidence that answers a focused clinical question with particular attention to the methodological quality of studies or the credibility of opinion and text. The JBI model takes a pluralistic approach to evidence synthesis that is inclusive of evidence that arises out of quantitative research; qualitative research; opinion; and economic analyses.

The synthesis of the results of quantitative research

Statistical analysis (meta-analysis) may or may not be used in synthesizing numerical data and this depends on the nature and quality of studies included in the review. Meta-analyses of numerical findings provide precise estimates of an association or a treatment effect in reviews of effectiveness through the statistical synthesis of multiple studies. Key outcomes of the meta-analysis are the measure of effect, the confidence interval, and the degree of heterogeneity of the studies synthesized.

The synthesis of the results of qualitative research

The term "meta-synthesis" refers to a "higher form of synthesis" or, as Light and Pillemer (1984) refer to it, the "science of summing up." Meta-synthesis is a process of combining the findings of individual qualitative studies (i.e., cases) to create summary statements that authentically describe the meaning of these themes.

The synthesis of evidence arising out of expert opinion and text

Although the proponents of evidence-based health care would argue that the results of high-quality research are the only source of evidence for practice, this has drawn considerable criticism from clinicians. Clinicians argue that the nature of everyday practice demands an eclectic, pragmatic approach to conceptualizing evidence. The "consumers" of systematic reviews – those who practice within the health system – regard the opinion of experts and the views of experienced clinicians and their professional bodies as valid forms of evidence for practice, especially when some intervention or activity is required in practice, even if no evidence from research exists. The process seeks to locate the major conclusions in text that represent credible opinion.

The synthesis of evidence arising out of economic analyses

The synthesis of economic analyses or evaluations is a developing science. The lack of standardization of systematic review methods is incongruous with the obvious need for these methods and the availability of existing effectiveness review methods that may be adapted in terms of searching, critical appraisal, and data extraction (Carande-Kulis *et al.*, 2000). Because of the paucity of high-quality studies and established methods to statistically synthesize studies meta-analysis is currently not widely used to synthesize economic findings; however, it is still obviously useful to extract data from high-quality studies and present a summation of the results in a way that informs practice. Syntheses of economic evidence can provide important information for health care decision makers and there is ongoing work that identifies "… the promise, difficulties, and current limitations of the use of economic analyses by healthcare decision makers" (Pignone *et al.*, 2005).

Evidence/knowledge transfer

This component of the model relates to the act of transferring knowledge to individual health professionals, health facilities, and health systems globally by means of journals, other publications, electronic media, education and training, and decision support systems. Evidence transfer is seen to involve more than disseminating or distributing information and to include careful development of strategies that identify target audiences – such as clinicians, managers, policy makers, and consumers – and designing methods to package and transfer information that is understood and used in decision making. Fundamental to this process is:

- Developing understandable and actionable messages.
- Accommodating the context of a target audience's information needs.
- Delivering messages in cost-effective ways (including information technology, print material, meetings, workshops, and training programs).

The model therefore depicts three major elements of evidence/knowledge transfer: education and training, information delivery, and the transfer of evidence though organizational and team systems.

Evidence Utilization

This component of the model relates the implementation of evidence in practice, as is evidenced by practice and/or system change. It identifies three elements: practice change; embedding evidence through system/organizational change; and evaluating the impact of the utilization of evidence on the health system, the process of care and health outcomes. Evidence utilization is highly influenced by factors such as resources, provider education/expertise, and patient preference as well as available research (Dicenso and Cullum, 1998). When the evidence suggest the use of a particular intervention and clinicians wish to implement such an intervention, to do so requires organizational planning and decision-making processes. Organizational factors, in addition to individual clinician factors, contribute to these problems; staffing levels and mix, the availability of consultation services, and policies are all examples of factors beyond the individual clinician's control (Nicklin and McVeety, 2002). Grimshaw *et al.* (2001), in a review of professional educational and quality assurance interventions, report that multifaceted interventions targeting different barriers to change are more likely to be effective than single interventions.

Intended users of the model

The JBI model was developed to convey the approach adopted by the JBI in the identification, synthesis, transfer, and utilization of evidence. This model has been used by the JBI's international network of centers and members to assist in the communication of what constitutes evidence, the usefulness of syntheses, and the process of dissemination and utilization of evidence to improve global health. The model is also used by health professionals to emphasize the importance of evidence informed practice; that evidence-based practice occurs when evidence is used with consideration of the context of care, the preference of the client, and the health professional's clinical judgment. The model is useful for teaching in both undergraduate and postgraduate contexts to demonstrate the cycle of evidence to inform practice derived from, and to benefit global health.

Hypotheses and propositions

The JBI model posits that implementing evidence-based health in any setting is *dependent upon* the generation of valid evidence; and *involves*:

- The synthesis of evidence (through searching for and appraising evidence).
- The transfer of evidence/knowledge to enable it to be accessed at the point-of-decision making (through disseminating summarized evidence and embedding evidence in information and decision-making systems).
- Implementing or utilizing evidence (through developing and pursuing strategies that generate, diffuse, and sustain practice change).

The model is linked to a collection of resources and tools to support the establishment of evidence-based practice (see Fig. 9.2).

The evidence utilization component of the model builds on the available international evidence on implementation science. A systematic review reported by the Centre for Reviews and Dissemination (1999) suggests that multiple interventions seem to be more effective than single interventions, but they conclude that implementation is complex. They go on to suggest that improving clinical effectiveness in health care requires the establishment of "… routine mechanisms by which individual and organisational change can occur" (Centre for Reviews and Dissemination, 1999: 1) and propose the

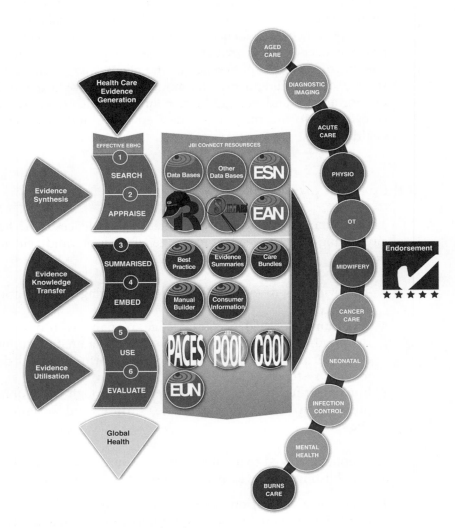

Figure 9.2 JBI resources and tools

following steps to be pursued in programs designed to transfer and utilize evidence:

- "A 'diagnostic analysis' to identify factors likely to influence the proposed change. Choice of dissemination and implementation interventions should be guided by the 'diagnostic analysis' and informed by knowledge of relevant research."
- "Multi-faceted interventions targeting different barriers to change are more likely to be effective than single interventions."
- "Any systematic approach to changing professional practice should include plans to monitor and evaluate, and to maintain and reinforce any change."

Of specific strategies found to be effective, audit and feedback appear to be promising (Thomson O'Brien *et al.*, 2000a, b); educational outreach (in the form of academic detailing) appears to have some positive effect in the area of prescribing (Thomson O'Brien *et al.*, 2002c); but continuing education does not appear to be effective (Thomson O'Brien *et al.*, 2001).

There is a growing literature that considers and/or evaluates specific processes of implementing evidence in practice. A robust evidence based on the feasibility, appropriateness, and meaningfulness of strategies to facilitate evidence utilization in health care is yet to be established. Grimshaw *et al.* (2001), in a review of professional education and quality assurance interventions, report that multifaceted interventions targeting different barriers to change are more likely to be effective than single interventions and Thomas *et al.* (1999) conclude from the findings of 18 studies that guideline-driven care can be effective in changing the process and outcome of care provided by professions allied to nursing. Kitson *et al.* (1996, 1998), Harvey *et al.*, 2002), and Rycroft-Malone *et al.* (2002) describe "The Promoting Action on Research Implementation in Health Services" (PARIHS) framework and its three key elements: the evidence, the context, and the facilitation. Others report on the role of guidelines and their dissemination in implementing change (Grimshaw *et al.*, 2004); the role of opinion leaders (Thomson O'Brien *et al.*, 2000d); and strategies to create a readiness for change and manage chan (Dzewaltowski *et al.*, 2004; Grol *et al.*, 2004).

The evidence utilization component of the JBI model this body of work to support a continuous evidence im cycle that involves making summarized evidence point-of-care; auditing practice using criteria that arise out of the evidence; identifying areas where practice is not consistent with the evidence and thus where there is a need for change; planning action to effect change; implementing the action; and repeating the audit to establish whether or not practice has improved (Fig. 9.3).

The "Practical Application of Clinical Evidence Systems"

The Practical Application of Clinical Evidence Systems (PACES) is a tool designed to be used alongside the JBI model. On the basis of an electronic training resource, the system consists of:

- A generic online database for the collection of data on a given activity or intervention whereby, based on the clinical audit process, data can be collected before and after a process of practice change as part of a continuous quality improvement (CQI) process.
- An online generic work plan (the "getting research into practice" – "GRIP" module) and related database related to problem identification, action planning, and action taking.

The program draws on approaches from the methodologies of clinical audit, participative action research, clinical leadership, and participative change management.

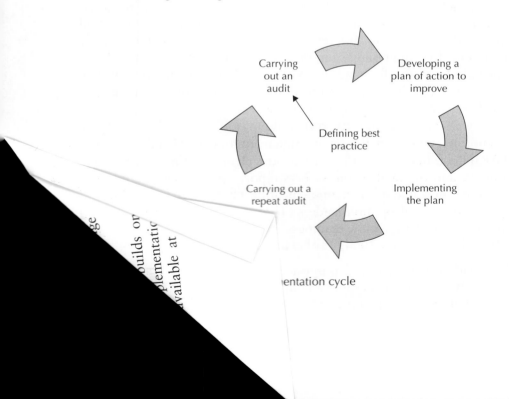

Clinical audit

Clinical audit is a process initiated and pursued by clinicians that seeks to improve the quality of care through structured peer review. The process involves clinicians in the examination of their practices and the outcomes of these practices against agreed standards and in changing practice when this is indicated. Essentially, "best practice" is identified and current practice is then surveyed and compared to agreed best practice. The results of the audit are then used to facilitate a process of change. The audit process is simply an organized way of deciding what should be (best practice); examining what is; and identifying the gaps between what should be and what is. Knowing the gaps, or the shortcomings in practice is the basis of the practice change cycle.

The "getting research into practice" module

Getting evidence from research into the everyday practices of health professionals to improve patient outcomes has yet to be (if ever) perfected. The aim of the GRIP module is to establish interprofessional processes within teams to examine barriers and facilitators to the utilization of evidence and design implementation programs to overcome the barriers identified. GRIP draws on the learning generated through the turning research into practice (TRIP) Initiative, commenced in 1999 by the then Agency for Health Care Policy and Research in the USA (now the AHRQ) to apply and assess strategies and methods developed in idealized practice settings or that were in current use but had not been previously or rigorously evaluated.

The GRIP module seeks to systematize approaches to the effective management of change to facilitate change within teams and consists of:

(1) Feeding back the audit results to all health professionals and service managers who are identified as stakeholders.
(2) Collecting naturalistic data from all stakeholders to elicit views on the validity of the standards and the evidence they are drawn from; the obstacles to implementing practice changes considered to be valid; and identifying possible strategies to overcome these barriers.
(3) Designing an implementation program based on steps 1 and 2.
(4) Conducting the implementation.

GRIP focuses on participative action and on the pursuit of knowledge through working collaboratively on describing the social world and acting on it to change it. Through acting on the world this way, critical understandings are generated. Participants in the process ask the question "What is happening here and how could it be different?" Consensual and participatory processes enable participants to set the agenda for change, and to prioritize issues they wish to focus on. GRIP fosters a process for participants to systematically investigate the problems and issues and to devise plans to deal with the problems at hand.

Leadership

The GRIP module emphasizes the role of clinical leaders. Clinical leaders – doctors, nurses, and allied health professionals – are seen to be central to the implementation of change and the achievement of excellence in others. Leadership has often been defined as a way of focusing and motivating a group to enable them to achieve their aims. It also involves being accountable and responsible for the group as a whole. Effective clinical leadership is identified as a key factor in implementing evidence in the JBI in evidence-based health care model; and understanding developing effective leadership skills in health care is, therefore, seen as fundamental to the utilization of evidence.

In a systematic review report on leadership in nursing *Pearson et al.* (2007) state that flexibility, trust, respect, support, consideration, and motivation are some of the characteristics of a leader that can result in positive outcomes and therefore a healthier work environment. Leaders who appeared to be effective were knowledgeable and educated as well as supportive and encouraging toward professional growth in their staff. Multiprofessional collaboration was also seen to be an important aspect of the leadership role. Communication is reported as a recurrent theme among the papers reviewed; leaders who communicated effectively and involved their staff in the decision-making process were seen as being involved in creating a healthy work environment.

Others' use of the JBI model for implementing evidence

The JBI model is in use in JBI collaborating health services in 47 countries, although the degree to which it has impacted on practice improvement and health outcomes has not yet been established. The model has, however, been applied over a 4-year period as part of the Evidence-Based Clinical Fellow project funded by the Australian Government Department of Health and Aging (both directly and more recently as part of the Encouraging Best Practice in Residential Aged Care Program [EBPRAC] initiative). Predicated on the view that, if the current focus on evidence-based practice is to lead to reductions in variability in practice and to an improvement in health outcomes, a strategy was needed to develop clinical leaders, and to assist provider agencies to refocus on developing clinical leaders with a sound understanding of the principles of best practice.

Contemporary approaches to the delivery of health care – including accreditation, audit, practice improvement, and a growing range of initiatives – focus on developing and using frameworks that identify "best practice." Use of these frameworks is facilitated through audit, quality management systems, and decision support for clinicians as they deliver care, and for managers, in their quality improvement role. The Evidence-Based Clinical Fellow project was designed to assist health professionals (nursing, allied health, or medicine) to acquire practical knowledge and skills in promoting best practice and in leading others in improving clinical practice, based on *the JBI model of evidence-based health care* and the use of the PACES and GRIP tools.

The aim of the Fellowship program was to introduce clinical leaders to change management and evidence-based practice processes and to help these leaders to become exemplars of how clinical leadership can be used to create and maintain a culture of clinical improvement.

Forty-nine participants completed the 6-month program between February 2005 and December 2008. Clinical Fellows participated in advanced education and training in the JBI model; practical approaches to identifying and using clinical evidence using the PACES and GRIP tools; and clinical leadership during an intensive training period of 5 days. They then returned to their practice area for 22 weeks to lead a process of change focusing on implementing evidence on a specific clinical topic using the JBI model and tools. During the fellowship period, advisors from the JBI gave regular telephone support and made an initial site visit to the Clinical Fellow's workplace prior to the intensive training period and a follow-up visit half way through the 24-week fellowship. Fellows spent another 5 days at the end of the fellowship at the JBI to finalize their report. All participants found the model appropriate and relevant; logical and understandable; and that the tools associated with model played a significant part in being able to generate practice change. All also report that they now use the model and the tools as part of their everyday, ongoing work.

All participating fellows successfully engaged in an action cycle of identifying best practice; auditing practice using criteria derived from evidence; fed back the audit results and established an action group; using the GRIP module, developed a plan of action; implemented the planned action; conducted a second audit; and compared the results of the pre- and post-action audits to establish if practice had improved and, if so, to what extent.

Grieve (2006) reports a significant improvement in the use of evidence-based care to prevent and manage constipation in adults; Georg (2006), Rivett (2006), and Keller (2006) conducted clinical audits using evidence-based criteria related to the maintenance of oral health and oral hydration and found significant improvements after implementing practice change. Similar outcomes are reported in the areas of medication administration (Bailey, 2008); the minimization of the use of physical restraint in a nursing home (Darcy, 2007); falls prevention (Fernandes, 2008; Gray *et al.*, 2008; Tran 2007); continence management (Heckenberg, 2008); and smoking cessation in young disabled clients (Nicholson, 2008).

Critique (strengths and weaknesses) of the JBI model for implementing evidence

The JBI model is neither an exhaustive model nor a tool kit for improving practice. The model provides a framework that continues to be developed and expanded by both the Institute and its collaborators to address the needs of health professionals to inform their practice with the best available research information.

The model is limited by the fact that it has been developed by the generators of evidence to inform health care practice. Health professionals, as users of evidence-based information will enter the cycle searching for summarized evidence in the form of systematic reviews or evidence summaries. Only if this summarized (synthesized) information is not available, primary research information is sought, which then requires critical appraisal and perhaps synthesis in the case of multiple studies being identified. A user engagement model was developed by the Institute in 2008 (JBI, 2008) (Fig. 9.4)

JBI Model for *User Engagement*
of Evidence-Based Information to infrom Clinical Decision Making

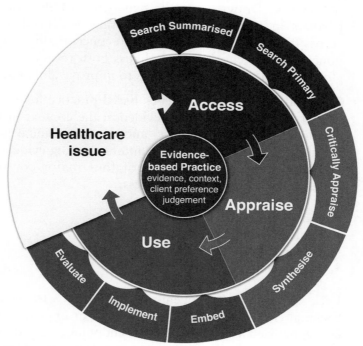

Figure 9.4 JBI model for user engagement

to represent the user approach to access (summarized and primary research), appraise (critically appraise and synthesize as appropriate), and use evidence (embed in practice systems, implement change, and evaluate outcomes) in response to health care issues.

Future plans

Implementing evidence will, like all change processes, always be challenging in health care. Investing in evidence-based practice through systematically reviewing the international evidence and producing and disseminating evidence summaries is not justifiable if a similar investment is not made to utilize the outputs of evidence reviews. Evidence-based health care is gaining acceptance globally. It is complex and sometimes misunderstood and frequently maligned. *The JBI model of evidence-based health care* has been constructed to enable reasoning and critique about evidence-based health care and its role in improving global health, within a logical conceptual framework. Drawn from the experience of the JBI and its global partners in promoting and facilitating evidence-based health care across the world, it is an attempt to conceptually represent the components of a cyclical process that is both responsive to priorities in global health and, in turn, serves to improve global health.

The model posits that evidence-based practice involves giving equal weight to the best available evidence; the context in which the care is delivered; client preference; and the professional judgment of the health professional. Promoting and facilitating evidence-based health care is depicted as consisting of four major components of the evidence-based health care process:

- Health care evidence generation.
- Evidence synthesis.
- Evidence/knowledge transfer.
- Evidence utilization.

Each of these components are modeled to incorporate three essential elements; and the achievement of improved global health is conceptualized as both the goal or endpoint of any or all of the model components and the *raison d'etre* and driver of evidence-based health care. Central to the model is a pluralistic approach to what constitutes legitimate evidence; an inclusive approach to evidence appraisal, extraction and synthesis; the importance of effective and appropriate transfer of evidence; and the complexity of evidence utilization.

Summary: How the model can be used/applied

As a framework for considering:

- What kind of research evidence can be used to inform practice?
- All research information should be critically appraised.
- When multiple, comparable studies are identified these should be synthesized.
- Disseminating information is distinct from the utilization of evidence.
- Implementation of evidence, whether within a single users practice or when embedded system wide, should be evaluated to establish impact on practice and client outcome.

Evidence implementation requires the use of multiple strategies and interventions, the JBI provide some tools that may be used by health professionals at the ward or organizational level to:
- identify and audit an area of practice using evidence-based criteria;
- develop, document, and implement a change strategy, engaging key stakeholders in the care setting;
- re-audit and compare results between audits;
- evaluate outcomes of the project.

References

Bailey, K. (2008). Medication administration in residential aged care. *PACEsetterS, 5*(3), 26.

Carande-Kulis, V.G., Maciosek, M.V., Briss, P.A., Teutsch, S.M., Zaza, S., Truman, B.I., Messonnier, M.L., Pappaioanou, M., Harris, J.R. and Fielding, J. (2000). Methods for systematic reviews of economic evaluations for the Guide to Community Preventive Services. Task Force on Community Preventive Services. *American Journal of Preventive Medicine*, 18(1 Suppl.), 75–91.

Centre for Reviews and Dissemination. (1999). Getting evidence into practice, *Effective Health Care, 5*, 1–16.

Darcy, L. (2007). Reducing and/or minimising physical restraint in a high care, rural aged care facility. *International Journal of Evidence-Based Healthcare, 5*(4), 458–467.

Dicenso, A. and Cullum, N. (1998). Implementing evidence-based nursing: Some misconceptions. *Evidence-based Nursing, 1*, 38–40.

Dzewaltowski, D.A., Glasgow, R.E., Klesges, L.M., Estabrooks, P.A., and Brock, E. (2004). RE-AIM: Evidence-based standards and a web resource to improve translation of research into practice. *Annals of Behavioral Medicine*, 28, 75–80.

Fernandes, G. (2008). Implementation of best practice in advance care planning in an 'ageing in place' aged care facility. *International Journal of Evidence-Based Healthcare*, 6(2), 270–276.

Georg, D. (2006). Improving the oral health of older adults with dementia/ cognitive impairment living in a residential aged care facility. *International Journal of Evidence-based Healthcare*, 4(1), 54–61.

Gray, L., McReynolds, T., and Jordan, Z. (2008). Falls prevention in a Secured Dementia Unit. *PACEsetterS, 5*(2), 14–15.

Grieve, J. (2006). The prevention and management of constipation in older adults in a residential aged care facility. *International Journal of Evidence-based Healthcare*, 4(1), 46–53.

Grimshaw, J.M., Shirran, L., Thomas, R.E., Mowatt, G., Fraser, C., Bero, L., Grilli, R., Harvey, E.L., Oxman, A.D., and O'Brien, M.A. (2001).

Changing provider behaviour: An overview of systematic reviews of interventions. *Medical Care*, 39(Suppl. 2), II-2–II-45.

Grimshaw, J.M., Thomas, R.E., MacLennan, G., *et al.* (2004). Effectiveness and efficiency of guideline dissemination and implementation strategies. *Health Technology Assessment*, 8(iii–iv), 1–72.

Grol, R., and Wensing, M. (2004). What drives change? Barriers to and incentives for achieving evidence-based practice. *Medical Journal of Australia*, 180(6 Suppl.), S57–S60.

Harvey, G., Loftus-Hills, A., Rycroft-Malone, J., *et al.* (2002). Getting evidence into practice: The role and function of facilitation. *Journal of Advanced Nursing*, 37, 577–588.

Heckenberg, G. (2008). Improving and ensuring best practice continence management in residential aged care. *International Journal of Evidence-Based Healthcare*, 6(2), 260–269.

Joanna Briggs Institute. (2008). JBI Message Strategy, Internal Discussion Paper 0908, September [unpublished internal document].

Keller, M. (2006). Maintaining oral hydration in older adults living in residential aged care facilities. *International Journal of Evidence-Based Healthcare*, 4(1), 68–73.

Kitson, A., Ahmed, L.B., Harvey, G., Seers, K., and Thompson, D.R. (1996). From research to practice: One organizational model for promoting research-based practice. *Journal of Advanced Nursing*, 23, 430–440.

Kitson, A., Harvey, G., and McCormack, B. (1998). Enabling the implementation of evidence-based practice a conceptual framework. *Quality in Health Care*, 7, 149–158.

Light, R.J. and Pillemer, D.B. (1984). *Summing Up: The Science of Reviewing Research*. Cambridge: Harvard University Press.

Miller, S. and Fredericks, M. (2003). The nature of "evidence" in qualitative research methods. *International Journal of Qualitative Methods*, 2(1). Article 4. Retrieved September 1, 2005 from http://www.ualberta.ca/~ijqm

Nicholson, E. (2008). Joanna Briggs Collaboration Aged Care Fellowship Project: Implementing a smoking cessation program in a young, frail aged residential care facility. *International Journal of Evidence-Based Healthcare*, 6(1), 111–118.

Nicklin, W. and McVeety, J. (2002). Canadian nurses describe their perceptions of patient safety in teaching hospitals. Wake up call! *Canadian Journal of Nursing Leadership* , 15, 11–21.

Pearson, A. (2004). Balancing the evidence: Incorporating the synthesis of qualitative data into systematic reviews. *JBI Reports*, 2(2), 45–64.

Pearson, A., Wiechula, R., Court, A., and Lockwood, C. (2005). The JBI model of evidence-based healthcare. *International Journal of Evidence-Based Healthcare*, 3(8), 207–215.

Pearson, A., Laschinger, H., Porritt, K., Jordan, Z., Tucker, D., and Long, L. (2007). Comprehensive systematic review of evidence on developing and sustaining nursing leadership that fosters a healthy work environment in healthcare. *International Journal of Evidence Based Healthcare, 5*(2), 208–253.

Pignone, M., Saha, S., Hoerger, T., and Mandelblatt, J. (2005). Cost-effectiveness analyses of colorectal cancer screening: A systematic review for the U.S. preventive services task force. *Annals of Internal Medicine, 137*(2), 96–104.

Rivett, D. (2006). Compliance with best practice in oral health: Implementing evidence in residential aged care. *International Journal of Evidence-Based Healthcare, 4*(1), 62–67.

Rycroft-Malone, J., Kitson, A., Harvey, G., McCormack, B., Seers, K., Titchen, A., and Estabrooks, C.A. (2002). Ingredients for change: Revisiting a conceptual framework. *Quality and Safety in Health Care, 11*, 174–180.

Thomas, L., Cullum, N., McColl, E., Rousseau, N., Soutter, J., and Steen, N. (1999). Guidelines in professions allied to medicine. *Cochrane Database of Systematic Reviews, 1*, CD000349. DOI: 10.1002/14651858. CD000349.

Thomson O'Brien, M.A., Oxman, A.D., Davis, D.A., Haynes, R.B., Freemantle, N., and Harvey, E.L. (2000a). Audit and feedback effects on professional practice and health care outcomes. *Cochrane Database of Systematic Reviews., 2*, CD000259.

Thomson O'Brien, M.A., Oxman, A.D., Davis, D.A., Haynes, R.B., Freemantle, N., and Harvey, E.L. (2000b). Audit and feedback versus alternative strategies effects on professional practice and health care outcomes. *Cochrane Database of Systematic Reviews, 2*, CD00260.

Thomson O'Brien, M.A., Oxman, A.D., Davis, D.A, Haynes, R.B., Freemantle, N., and Harvey, E.L. (2000c). Educational outreach visits effects on professional practice and health care outcomes. *Cochrane Database of Systematic Reviews, 2*, CD000409.

Thomson O'Brien, M.A., Oxman, A.D., Haynes, R.B., Davis, D.A., Freemantle, N., and Harvey, E.L. (2000d). Local opinion leaders effects on professional practice and health care outcomes. *Cochrane Database of Systematic Reviews Syst Rev, 2*, CD000125. [PubMed]

Thomson O'Brien, M.A., Freemantle, N., Oxman, A.D., Wolf, F., Davis, D.A., and Herrin, J. (2001). Continuing education meetings and workshops effects on professional practice and health care outcomes. *Cochrane Database of Systematic Reviews, 2*, CD03030.

Tran, T. (2007). Implementing best practice in identifying falls risk among the elderly in a residential care setting. *PACEsetterS, 4*(4), 16–21.

Chapter 10

The Knowledge To Action framework

Ian D Graham and Jacqueline M Tetroe

Key learning points

- The Knowledge To Action (KTA) framework, based on a concept analysis of 31 planned action theories, was developed to help make sense of the black box known as "knowledge translation" or "implementation" by offering a holistic view of the phenomenon by integrating the concepts of knowledge creation and action.
- The framework assumes a systems perspective, and falls within the social constructivist paradigm which privileges social interaction and adaptation of research evidence, taking local context and culture into account.
- It was designed to be used by a broad range of audiences and has been widely cited, but has not, as yet, been tested empirically.
- While the framework does not specifically prescribe what needs to be done at each phase, the set of 31 theories on which the framework is based, can provide more specific guidance.
- Future iterations of the KTA cycle will be informed by feedback from the researchers and knowledge-users who are trying to apply it.

There are two kinds of science: applied and not yet applied.

—George Porter, former president of Britain's Royal Society

This chapter describes the conceptual framework for knowledge translation (KT) that is known as the Knowledge To Action (KTA) process (Graham and Tetroe, 2007b; Graham *et al.*, 2006). This framework provides a map to guide the application of knowledge – to move not-yet-applied science into the realm of the applied. Figure 10.1 illustrates the framework.

Purpose of the framework

Conceptual frameworks have the basic purpose of focusing, ruling some things in as relevant and ruling others out because of their lesser importance. Their usefulness comes from the organization they provide for thinking, for observation, and for interpreting what is seen. They provide a systematic structure and a rationale for activities. In general, conceptual frameworks are made up of concepts and propositions designed to focus the user on what is important to the

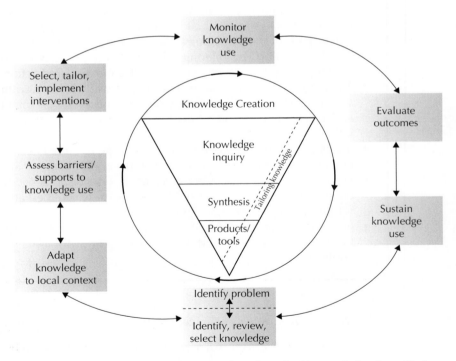

Figure 10.1 The Knowledge To Action cycle (adapted with permission from Graham *et al.,* 2006)

issue (Rimmer and Johnson Lutjens, 1998). The KTA framework was developed to help make sense of the black box known as "knowledge translation" or "implementation" by offering a holistic view of the phenomenon by integrating the concepts of knowledge creation and action. Given that the action component of the framework was derived from a synthesis of planned action models, the KTA process may be considered a planned action model in that it directs attention to the ideal phases or categories of action that are believed to be important when attempting to implement change.

Assumptions

The ultimate aim of KTA is improved health and health care. The KTA framework, like all planned action theories, assumes a systems perspective. In the field of health, knowledge producers and users are situated within a social system or systems that are responsive and adaptive, although not always in predictable ways. Therefore, the KTA process is considered iterative, dynamic, and complex, both concerning knowledge creation and knowledge application (action cycle), with the boundaries between the creation and action components and their ideal phases being fluid and permeable. The action phases may occur sequentially or simultaneously and the knowledge phases may influence or be drawn upon during action phases. The cyclic nature of the process and the critical role of feedback loops are key concepts that underlie our conceptual model. While knowledge can be empirically derived (i.e., research based) the framework encompasses other forms of knowing such as contextual and experiential knowledge as well. The framework falls within the social constructivist paradigm and privileges social interaction and adaptation of research evidence that takes local context and culture into account as key mechanisms necessary for turning knowledge into action.

Another fundamental aspect of the framework is that it is designed to accommodate both end of project and integrated KT (Graham and Tetroe, 2007a, 2008; Tetroe, 2007). With the end of project KT, the knowledge producers (typically researchers) create the knowledge and the knowledge users focus exclusively on the uptake of the new knowledge with the two activities carried out sequentially and therefore in isolation of each other with little direct interaction between the knowledge producers and users. Within the framework the knowledge creation and action components can be "activated" by different stakeholders and groups (working independently of each other at different points in time). In contrast, integrated KT represents a different way of doing research and involves active collaboration between researchers and knowledge users throughout the research and action/application process. This approach/concept has also been referred to as collaborative (Denis and Lomas, 2003; Lomas, 2000), participatory, or action-oriented research (Macaulay *et al.*, 1999); community-based research (Minkler and Wallerstein, 2003); copro- duction of knowledge or Mode 2 knowledge production (Gibbons *et al.*, 1994). When the framework is taken as a whole it can represent knowledge producers and knowledge users working collaboratively throughout the KTA process.

Adherence to each phase of the framework is not sufficient itself to ensure the successful application of knowledge. A key assumption underlying the framework is the importance of appropriate relation- ships – between researchers and knowledge-users; between imple- menters and adopters; and between the targeted groups and subgroups of adopters. Therefore, it is implicit within the framework that the roles of researchers and knowledge users would be less distinct than usual, laying the foundation for the proposition that researchers, prac- titioners, and decision makers need to sort out their perspective roles throughout the process.

Background and context

The origins of the KTA process can be traced to a research project funded by the Canadian Institutes of Health Research in 2004. The study involved undertaking a synthesis of planned action or change theories/models in the health sciences, social sciences, education, and management fields. A planned change model/theory is a set of logi- cally interrelated concepts that explain, in a systematic way, the means by which planned change occurs, that predict how various forces in an environment will react in specified change situations, and that help planners or change agents control variables that increase or decrease the likelihood of the occurrence of change (Rimmer and Johnson Lutjens, 1998; Tiffany, 1994; Tiffany and Lutjens, 1998; Tiffany *et al.*, 1994). Planned action/change, in this context, refers to deliberately engineering change that occurs in groups that vary in size and setting. Planned change models/theories are also referred to as prescriptive models/theories. Those who use planned change models/theories may work with individuals, but their objective is to alter ways of doing things in social systems.

Focused electronic searches for planned action or change theories yielded 3840 articles and 144 dissertation references. An Internet search identified an additional 103 documents and hand searching key journals identified another 142 potential papers of interest. From this we identified 31 planned action theories published between 1983 and 2006 which were subjected to a theory analysis. Two reviewers independently abstracted key or core concepts of each model/theory, determining the action phases and deciding whether each fit the inclusion/exclusion criteria around being a planned action model/theory. All the components of each model/theory were examined to determine commonalities and to develop a framework to be able to compare each of them. This sifting exercise resulted in 16 action steps that were reduced to 10 actions steps, which were subsequently reduced again into 7 phases in the action cycle (see discussion and Table 10.1 in the following text).

Table 10.1 Phases and constructs comprising the Knowledge To Action process

Phases	Constructs
Identify problem/identify, review, select knowledge ($n = 29$)	Identify a problem that needs addressing ($n = 19$ planned action theories) Identify the need for change ($n = 22$) Identify change agents (i.e., the appropriate actors to bring about the change) ($n = 15$) Identify target audience ($n = 13$) Review evidence/literature ($n = 21$)
Adapt knowledge to local context ($n = 11$)	Develop/adapt innovation ($n = 11$)
Assess barriers to knowledge use ($n = 18$)	Assess barriers to using the knowledge ($n = 18$)
Select, tailor, implement interventions ($n = 28$)	Select and tailor interventions to promote the use of the knowledge ($n = 26$) Link to appropriate individuals or groups who have vested interests in the project ($n = 11$) Pilot test ($n = 11$) Implement ($n = 22$)
Monitor knowledge use ($n = 14$)	Develop a plan to evaluate use of the knowledge ($n = 14$)
Evaluate outcomes ($n = 23$)	Evaluate the process ($n = 19$) Evaluate the outcomes ($n = 20$)
Sustain knowledge use ($n = 11$)	Maintain change – sustain ongoing knowledge use ($n = 11$) Disseminate results of the implementation process ($n = 7$)

n, number of planned action theories with this phase/construct. Total number of theories analyzed $n = 31$.

At around the same time, two members of the team (IDG, JT) were asked to consult with Health Canada on developing a framework to assess the impact of Federal research investments in HIV/AIDS. While seeing the potential value of proposing an action cycle based on the synthesis that had been undertaken, it also became clear that the application of existing research by knowledge users was the focus of many of the planned action/change models. While the action phases represent a process, they require *content* to be operationalized and knowledge creation, synthesis and the application of tools comprise the knowledge (or content) to be moved to action. Through reflection, debate, and from feedback on evolving presentations at grand rounds, academic meetings, and conferences, the final version of the KTA process emerged. Given the action cycle's grounding in planned action theory, the framework can be considered evidence-informed.

Framework description

In the depiction of the KTA process (Fig. 10.1), the triangle/funnel symbolizes knowledge creation and the cycle represents the activities or processes related to application of knowledge (usually requiring action by the potential users of the knowledge).

Knowledge creation

Knowledge creation, or the production of knowledge, is composed of three phases: knowledge inquiry (first-generation knowledge), knowledge synthesis (second-generation knowledge), and creation of knowledge tools and/or products (third-generation knowledge). The knowledge funnel/triangle in the figure represents a knowledge sieve. As knowledge is filtered or distilled through each stage in the knowledge creation process, the resulting knowledge becomes more synthesized and potentially more useful to end users. For example, the synthesis stage attempts to identify common patterns by bringing together the disparate research findings that may exist globally on a topic. At the tools/products development stage, the highest quality knowledge and research is further synthesized and distilled into decision-making tools such as practice guidelines, algorithms, or decision aids.

Action cycle

The seven action phases can occur sequentially or simultaneously and the knowledge funnel can be brought to bear on the action phases at several points in the cycle. At each phase there are multiple theories from different disciplines which can be drawn upon to guide the process. Included are the processes needed to implement knowledge in health and health care settings namely identification of the problem or identifying, reviewing, and selecting the knowledge to implement; adapting or customizing the knowledge to the local context; assessing the determinants of knowledge use; selecting, tailoring, implementing, and monitoring KT interventions and use of the knowledge; evaluating outcomes or impact of using the knowledge, and determining strategies for ensuring sustained knowledge use.

The action phases enable the framing of what needs to be done, how, and what circumstances/conditions need to be addressed when implementing change. They are not meant to replace or override the component theories from which the phases were derived. For example, when addressing the barriers to knowledge use, 18 of the 31 planned action theories had a construct dealing with this – some with more precision and coverage than others. Furthermore, for each action phase other (nonplanned action) theories (psychological, organizational, economic, sociological, educational, etc.) may be relevant and useful (see, e.g., Wensing *et al.*, 2009).

Table 10.1 presents the action phases as well as the subconstructs comprising each that were derived from the synthesis of planned action theories. The table indicates how many planned action theories included the phase or subconstructs of the phase. While 16 unique constructs were identified, they were "rolled up" into the 7 phases that appear in the model, based on the considerable implementation experience of the research team and on the goal of developing an elegant, usable model that would resonate with potential users by balancing practicality and level of detail. The 16 constructs in some cases provide substeps of the phases and in other cases they are the same as the phase. For example, we saw the five constructs that comprise the phase "identify the problem/identify, review, selec" knowledge" as a critical but collective first step of the KTA proc While the component constructs are distinct, we saw them a part of one phase. On the other hand, the phase: "adapt k to local context" maps directly on to the construct: "de innovation." No other constructs emerged from the concept analyses that were operationally similar.

The dotted cycle circling the knowledge creation component (see Fig. 10.1) is intended to illustrate that at each phase of the action cycle one should consider its role (including knowledge inquiry, synthesis, or tools and products). Each phase could be informed and guided by the relevant knowledge base, where one exists, and the results of implementation work undertaken could also inform the knowledge base.

The planned action theory action constructs (as discussed in the preceding text) were always described within a context or via examples that were defined within a specific context. As a result of this, the team developed a set of contextual factors that were used to code each of the action phases in order to capture the subtle distinctions of constructs from one planned action theory to another. These contextual factors included the following.

(1)   Nature of the evidence/knowledge – does it justify the innovation? Is it compelling to the target audience?
(2)   Attributes of the change/innovation – is the innovation suitable to be implemented in this setting, is it consistent with identified values, goals, needs, etc.?
(3)   Audience – concern of various audiences about different aspects of the implementation process.
(4)   Context/culture – the physical, social, and organizational aspects of the implementation environment.
(5)   Resources/support – are there sufficient resources (including human resources) for the innovation?
(6)   Implementation-related factors – strategies or factors that facilitate the implementation of the intervention.

These f   ganizational in nature and are the context in
                    ses operate. Seeing the action categories within
                    ntext has always been our approach to under-
                    cess. While the representation of the cycle may
                    plexity, our framework is actually a dynamic
                    would argue that, while this representation
                    a sequence of phases that need to be taken in
                    implementation projects unfold in "real life."
                    , and move forward in an erratic manner with
                    ections as the action phases accommodate the
                    haps a better representation of our framework

would be the probabilistic atomic model, where the action phases are like electrons around the nucleus of knowledge generation – and the contextual factors influence where a given phase might be at a specific time.

Intended audiences/users

The KTA framework was designed to be used by a broad range of audiences. Because it is the result of a synthesis of planned action theories, it was not conceived within a specific context, with a particular audience in mind. The original planned action theories were targeted to bring about change for variety of audiences: Most frameworks were targeted to: practitioners ($n = 29$), administrators/ managers ($n = 25$), policy makers ($n = 15$), although many were also designed to be useful to researchers ($n = 12$), patients ($n = 7$), and the public ($n = 3$). Many of the theories were targeted to more than one audience. Similarly, of all the theories, the intended purpose for 27 of them was to guide practice, while 7 were designed to guide research and 5 to guide theory. The KTA framework is appropriate for use with individuals, teams, or organizations working in diverse contexts.

In January 2009, we conducted a Google Scholar search for citations of the original "Lost in Knowledge Translation" paper and found around 50 unique citations (we know of more that were not yet picked up by the search engine). The titles of the articles, reports, theses, or book chapters citing this article suggested that the framework was being used both for advancing/discussing the science of KT and to guide change in both practice and policy. The articles cited were written by or targeted to a broad array of audiences: policy makers, researchers, and individuals, teams, and organizations within the health professions.

Hypotheses and research possibilities – Has the framework generated hypotheses or propositions that the developers and others can and/or have been testing?

To our knowledge, the framework has not been tested empirically, but there are a number of hypotheses or propositions that can be generated from the KTA cycle that could be tested. The most obvious hypothesis is that application of all components of the framework will distinguish more from less successful implementation projects. Similarly, adoption of an integrated approach to KT should be more effective than the approach in which researchers produce knowledge in a vacuum, without continuous collaboration with knowledge-users. The relative contribution of each of the phases to the success of an implementation project needs to be investigated. For example, how important is it to adapt knowledge to a local context? If it is important, what is the best process to use to accomplish this? Furthermore, hypotheses can be generated about the specific knowledge and skill sets required for successful management of each of the phases.

The importance of the context embedded in the KTA cycle would suggest that organizational cultures that favor evidence-informed planning/decision making and resource allocation are more likely to successfully implement intended changes. But even in organizations that apply the framework, there may be differential success in achieving sustainable implementation without an identified and designated change agent to enact it – to move the framework itself into action.

Evaluation and use of the KTA framework

We are unaware of studies that have been specifically designed to evaluate the KTA framework. However, at the time we conducted our theories analysis, 10 of the theories (DiCenso *et al.*, 2002; Doyle *et al.*, 2001; Feifer and Ornstein, 2004; Graham and Logan, 2004; Green and Kreuter, 1999; Herie and Martin, 2002; Rosswurm and Larrabee, 1999; Stetler, 2003; Titler *et al.*, 2001; Tracy *et al.*, 2006), had been empirically tested. Furthermore, a bibliometric analysis of the component theories conducted at the time our framework was initially derived indicated that uptake varied from one theory to another. The mean number of citations for each theory was 32, ranging from 1 to 173.

Our Google Scholar search for citations of the KTA framework indicates that despite it only being published in 2006, there is wide awareness of it, with citations in over 25 journals, including nursing, specialist health journals, health policy, and generalist journals such as the Lancet and the BMJ. It was also referenced in a number of dissertations, book chapters, and web-based reports. The framework has become a key part of messaging about KT at CIHR since September 2007. It has been presented to a variety of CIHR's stakeholders and internal staff, and has been well received in the sense that it is understandable and relatively simple, yet comprehensive. Many of the proposals submitted to the funding opportunities offered by the KT portfolio at CIHR reference or explicitly use the framework to guide and evaluate their work. The Canadian Partnerships Against Cancer (Kerner, 2009) has adapted the framework to guide their knowledge management strategy. Finally, the K2A cycle has also been used as a framework for the KT Clearinghouse (http:// ktclearinghouse.ca/), a repository of KT tools and resources and as a way to organize the chapters in an edited book about KT (Straus *et al.*, 2009).

Strengths and limitations

A number of strengths of the KTA process have been noted including: the model integrates knowledge creation and action and is explicitly-grounded in planned action theory; it focuses on local context and practice when adapting and implementing evidence-informed interventions (practices, programs, policies); it assumes the participation/ engagement of knowledge users in: producing the knowledge, adapting it for use, and selecting and tailoring implementation interventions to their context; it recognizes that knowledge may not be entirely research based, allowing for the blending of contextual knowledge in selecting the research and the implementation interventions to apply; it focuses on two-way interaction and communications between knowledge producers and users throughout the discovery–application cycle and the reintegration of foundational research with implementation research; it distinguishes between monitoring knowledge use and evaluating the impact of using the knowledge. Feedback from researchers and knowledge users suggests that the KTA process provides a useful way of thinking about KT but more importantly, by breaking the process into manageable pieces, it provides a structure and rationale for activities.

The framework does not however prescribe specifically what needs to be done at each phase in the process nor populate each phase with mid and micro range theory which might direct action at each phase. Indeed, other social, psychological, educational, organizational, economic, theories can be incorporated into each of the frameworks constructs. However, the set of 31 theories on which the framework is based, can provide more specific guidance for each phase. Furthermore, the two-dimensional, linear representation of the framework might seem to preclude the possibility that change can occur at multiple levels, but not necessarily at the same pace and that there is a need for coordination and communication to align and shepherd these change processes. While not explicitly stated, there is nothing inherent about the framework that would exclude its use at multiple levels. Ferlie *et al.* (2005) cite the work of Van de Ven *et al.* (1999) and others that confirm nonlinear models of innovation spread. They argue that there is no linear flow or prescribed sequence of stages. "Indeed, flow is a radically inappropriate image to describe what are erratic, circular, or abrupt processes, which may come to a full stop or go into reverse" (Ferlie *et al.*, 2005: 123). The KTA cycle, despite its two-dimensional representation does not preclude this description of the change process. The one other potential limitation is that the KTA framework does require a stable and responsive research agenda and platform (required structures and resources) to support close collaboration between researchers and knowledge users which may not be in place in many contexts.

Future plans for the development of the framework

Future iterations of the KTA cycle will be informed by feedback from the researchers and knowledge-users who are trying to apply it. We intend to follow up with CIHR-funded researchers who used the model in their applications to determine how effective it was in guiding/evaluating the application of knowledge; we also intend to determine its utility as a classification system/schema for CIHR-funded integrated KT projects – whether or not they explicitly used the framework. We have the unique advantage of having a funding agency use our framework and we can now assess the degree and effectiveness of its uptake.

Summary: How the model can be used/applied

- Given that the framework was derived from a synthesis of planned action models, the KTA process directs attention to the ideal phases or categories of action that are believed to be important when attempting to implement change *in any setting*.
- It can be used for both "end of grant" and "integrated" KT endeavors.

- The KTA framework is appropriate for use with individuals, teams, or organizations working in diverse contexts.
- The framework has been cited by articles targeting a broad array of audiences: policy makers, researchers, and individuals, teams, and organizations within the health professions.
- It has also been used as an organizing framework for a book and a website "clearing house" on KT.

References

Best, A., Terpstra, J., and Moor, G. (2008). *Conceptual Frameworks for Knowledge to Action.*

Denis, J.L. and Lomas, J. (2003). Convergent evolution: The academic and policy roots of collaborative research. *Journal of Health Services Research and Policy,* 8(Suppl. 2), 1–6.

DiCenso, A., Virani, T., Bajnok, I., Borycki, E., Davies, B., Graham, I., *et al.* (2002). A toolkit to facilitate the implementation of clinical practice guidelines in healthcare settings. *Hospital Quarterly, 5,* 55–60.

Doyle, D.M., Dauterive, R., Chuang, K.H., and Ellrodt, A.G. (2001). Translating evidence into practice: Pursuing perfection in pneumococcal vaccination in a rural community. *Respiratory Care, 46,* 1258–1272.

Feifer, C. and Ornstein, S. (2004). Strategies for increasing adherence to clinical guidelines and improving patient outcomes in small primary care practices. *Joint Commission Journal on Quality and Safety, 30,* 432–431.

Ferlie, E., Fitzgerald, L., Wood, M., and Hawkins, C. (2005). The nonspread of innovations: The mediating role of professionals. *Academy of Management Journal, 48,* 117–134.

Gibbons, M., Limoges, C., Nowotny, H., Schwartzmann, S., Scott, P., and Trow, M. (1994). *The New Production of Knowledge: The Dynamics of Science and Research in Contemporary Societies.* London: Sage.

Graham, I.D. and Logan, J. (2004). Innovations in knowledge transfer and continuity of care. *Canadian Journal of Nursing Research, 36,* 89–103.

Graham, I.D. and Tetroe, J. (2007a). How to translate health research knowledge into effective healthcare action. *Healthcare Quarterly, 10,* 20–22.

Graham, I.D. and Tetroe, J. (2007b). Some theoretical underpinnings of knowledge translation. *Academic Emergency Medicine, 14,* 936–941.

Graham, I.D. and Tetroe, J. (2008). Nomenclature in translational research. *JAMA, 299,* 2149–2150.

Graham, I.D., Logan, J., Harrison, M.B., Straus, S., Tetroe, J.M., Caswell, W., *et al.* (2006). Lost in knowledge translation: Time for a map? *Journal of Continuing Education in Health Professions, 26,* 13–24.

Green, L.W. and Kreuter, M.W. (1999). *Health Promotion Planning: An Educational and Ecological Approach* (3rd edn). Mountain View, CA: Mayfield Publishing Company.

Herie, M. and Martin, G.W. (2002). Knowledge diffusion in social work: A new approach to bridging the gap. *Social Work, 47,* 85–95.

Kerner, J. (2009). Knowledge translation in cancer surveillance: What do we know, how should we share it, and who cares? Canadian Partnership against Cancer.

Lomas, J. (2000). Using "linkage and exchange" to move research into policy at a Canadian foundation. *Health Affairs, 19,* 236–240.

Macaulay, A.C., Commanda, L.E., Freeman, W.L., Gibson, N., McCabe, M.L., Robbins, C.M., *et al.* (1999). Participatory research maximises community and lay involvement. North American Primary Care Research Group. *BMJ, 319,* 774–778.

Minkler, M. and Wallerstein, N. (2003). *Community-Based Participatory Research for Health.* San Francisco, CA: Jossey-Bass Inc.

Rimmer, T.C. and Johnson Lutjens, L.R. (1998). *Planned Change Theories for Nursing. Review, Analysis and Implications.* Thousand Oaks, CA: Sage.

Rosswurm, M.A. and Larrabee, J.H. (1999). A model for change to evidence-based practice. *Image: Journal of Nursing Scholarship, 31,* 317–322.

Stetler, C. (2003). Updating the Stetler Model of research use to facilitate evidence-based practice. *Nursing Outlook, 24,* 272–279.

Straus, S., Tetroe, J.M., and Graham, I.D. (2009). *Knowledge Translation in Health Care: Moving from Evidence to Practice.* London: Wiley-Blackwell.

Tetroe, J. (2007). *Knowledge Translation at the Canadian Institutes of Health Research: A Primer* (Rep. No. Technical Brief No. 18). National Center for the Dissemination of Disability Resreach (NCDDR).

Tiffany, C. (1994). Analysis of planned change theories. *Nursing Management, 25,* 60–62.

Tiffany, C. and Lutjens, L. (1998). *Planned Change Theories for Nursing. Review, Analysis, and Implications.* Thousand Oaks, CA: Sage Publications.

Tiffany, C., Cheatham, A., Doornbos, D., Loudermelt, L., and Momadi, G. (1994). Planned change theory: Survey of nursing periodical literature. *Nursing Management, 25,* 54–59.

Titler, M.G., Kleiber, C., Steelman, V., Rakel, B., Budreau, G., Everett, L.N., *et al.* (2001). The Iowa Model of evidence-based practice to promote quality care. *Critical Care Nursing Clinics of North America, 13,* 497–509.

Tracy, S., Dufault, M., Kogut, S., Martin, V., Rossi, S., and Willey-Temkin, C. (2006). Translating best practices in nondrug postoperative pain management. *Nursing Research, 55,* S57–S67.

Van de Ven, A., Polley, D., Garud, R., and Venkataraman, S. (1999). *The Innovation Journey*. Oxford, England: Oxford University Press.

Wensing, M., Bosch, M., and Grol, R. (2009). Selecting, tailoring and implementing knowledge translation interventions. In: S. Straus, J.M. Tetroe, and Graham I.D. (eds), *Knowledge Translation in Health Care: Moving from Evidence to Practice* (pp. 94–112). London: Wiley-Blackwell.

Chapter 11

Analysis and synthesis of models and frameworks

Jo Rycroft-Malone and Tracey Bucknall

Background

This chapter synthesizes some of the key features of the models and frameworks described in the previous chapters. To arrive at this summary, we read each chapter and made a judgment about the frameworks and models based on the description the developers had given us and using a number of dimensions that included:

- Type
- Purpose
- Development
- Theoretical underpinnings
- Conceptual clarity
- Levels
- Situation
- Users
- Function
- Testable.

These dimensions and their subdimensions were created from evidence about theory and framework robustness described in Chapter 2. The first five dimensions relate to the framework or models' development and conceptual underpinning (Table 11.1), the remaining five dimensions relate more specifically to their use (Table 11.2). While we have applied these criteria to the models and frameworks in this

Table 11.1 Assessment of models and frameworks on development criteria

Model	Type		Purpose			Development		Theoretical underpinning		Conceptual clarity
	Model	Framework	Descriptive	Explanatory	Predictive	Inductive	Deductive	Implicit	Explicit	
Stetler	x		x	x		x			x	x
OMRU (Ottowa)	x		x	x		x			x	x
PARIHS		x	x	x		x			x	x
Iowa	x		x	x			x	x		
Dobbins		x	x		x		x		x	x
ARCC		x	x			x			x	
JBI	x		x			x		x		x
KTA		x	x	x	x	x	x		x	x

PARIHS, Promoting Action on Research Implementation in Health Services; ARCC, Advancing Research and Clinical practice through close Collaboration; JBI, Joanna Briggs Institute; KTA, Knowledge To Action; OMRU, Ottowa Model for Research Use.

Table 11.2 Assessment of models and frameworks on application criteria

Models	Levels				Situation			Users					Function				
	Individual	Team	Unit	Organization	Policy	Hypothetical	Real	Nurses	Medics	Allied health	Multidisciplinary	Policy makers	Assessment of facilitators and barriers	Intervention/ strategy development	Outcome measurement and variable selection	Evaluation of process	Testable
Stetler	×	×	×				×	×					×	×	×	×	×
OMRU (Ottowa)	×	×	×	×			×	×	×	×	×		×	×	×	×	×
PARIHS		×	×	×	×		×	×	×	×	×		×	×		×	×
Iowa	×	×	×	×		×	×	×	×	×	×			×	×	×	×
Dobbins				×	×	×	×	×	×	×	×	×	×	×		×	×
ARCC	×			×			×	×				×	×	×			×
JBI			×	×			×	×					×	×		×	
KTA	×	×	×	×	×		×	×	×	×	×	×	×	×	×	×	×

PARIHS, Promoting Action on Research Implementation in Health Services; ARCC, Advancing Research and Clinical practice through close Collaboration; JBI, Joanna Briggs Institute; KTA, Knowledge To Action; OMRU, Ottowa Model for Research Use.

book, our intention is for them to be used to assess *any* model or framework's robustness and applicability.

Our intention is not to make a value judgment about each of the models or frameworks, but to provide the reader with a resource to help determine which of them might be appropriate in particular circumstances. As such, what we have done is provide a narrative summary of how the frameworks and models relate to each of the dimensions. The remainder of the chapter is structured around these dimensions and considers the implications for use. Chapter 12 provides a summary, and specific application examples.

Synthesis

Table 11.1 provides an illustration of how each framework and model featured on each of the dimensions. Essentially, the presence of an x means that the particular feature or attribute is present and/or relevant; a judgment made based on the information the model and framework developers have provided. For example, one of our criteria is about whether the model or framework is applicable at an individual, team, unit, organization, and/or policy level. The presence of a x in these columns means that the particular model is relevant at one (or more) of these levels. The following sections provide a detailed analysis and discussion of our findings.

Type

Using the definitions we presented in Chapter 2, we used the following criteria to make a judgment about whether each heuristic is a model or a framework:

- A framework can provide anything from a skeletal set of variables to something as extensive as a paradigm. They are made up of a set of concepts, and the relationships between the concepts such that they facilitate the development of propositions (i.e., about the relationships between the concepts in the framework). Their purpose is in providing a frame of reference, for organizing thinking, as a guide for what to focus on, and for interpretation.
- A model is more precise and more prescriptive than a framework. The concepts within them should be well defined and the relationships between the concepts more defined. Models are

representations of the real thing; they attempt to objectify the concept they represent.

As Table 11.1 shows, the previous chapters have explained a mixture of both models and frameworks. The following are characterized as models:

- Stetler model,
- Ottawa Model of Research Use (OMRU),
- Iowa model for EBP
- Dobbins *et al.'s* dissemination and use of research evidence for policy and practice model, and
- Advancing Research and Clinical practice through close Collaboration (ARCC) model,

and the following as conceptual frameworks:

- Promoting Action on Research Implementation in Health Services (PARIHS),
- the Joanna Briggs Institute (JBI) model of evidence-based health care as a framework for implementing evidence, and
- the Knowledge To Action (KTA) framework.

To a certain extent, these labels have been determined by the developers as a result of how they name their particular model or framework, and described in more detail in the previous chapters. When considering the definitions of frameworks and models that were developed from the literature about theory and outlined above, the extent to which these heuristics meet these criteria vary. For example, the models in the above list show varying degrees of specificity or preciseness. The Stetler model, perhaps by virtue of the fact that it has been in development for many years and has been through several iterations is relatively precise and prescriptive as a planned action theory. Similarly, the Ottawa Model of Research Use is precise, but perhaps less prescriptive than the Stetler model; while the overall processes and components of research use are detailed, there is perhaps more flexibility within each of them. In contrast, Dobbins *et al.'* dissemination and use of research evidence for policy and practice model, is less precise and prescriptive. However, their definition of models and frameworks differs to ours,' which likely accounts for the difference in our categorization. Melnyk and Fineout-Overholt in their description of the ARCC model, describe it as an "organized conceptual framework to guide system wide implementation and sustainability of EBP ...." While there are elements of prescription, there is also some flexibility within the ARCC model. The same is the case for the Iowa model for evidence-based practice (EBP) to promote quality care; there are sequences and prompts at each stage, however there is latitude within each of these, that is, it is not prescriptive.

In contrast to the models, the frameworks included within this book are less prescriptive, but provide readers with the sort of things that need to be paid attention to within implementation work. For example, the PARIHS framework represents implementation as a function of the three broad concepts; nature of the *evidence*, the quality of the *context* of evidence use, and the way in which implementation processes are *facilitated*. The Knowledge To Action framework offers a holistic view of the integration of the concepts of knowledge creation (knowledge inquiry, synthesis, products/tools, and particularization) and action (planned action theory). The JBI model of evidence-based health care is an overarching framework for EBP that includes four main components; evidence generation, evidence synthesis, evidence/knowledge transfer, and evidence use.

The difference between the models and frameworks outlined in the preceding text and described in detail in earlier chapters is in their level of preciseness and attention to the processes of implementation. The three frameworks provide more of a conceptual map of the factors that need to be accounted for when implementing evidence into practice. In contrast, the models provide more specific detail on the processes and stages one could use to implement evidence into practice. Of course there is no reason why the use of a framework could not be combined with the use of a more process-oriented model. Some of the other potential uses of the various frameworks and models are considered throughout this chapter, and summarized in Chapter 12.

Purpose

Linked to the literature about theory we were interested in understanding what the models and frameworks could offer in the way of description, explanation, and prediction, where the following were used as criteria:

- *Descriptive:* The framework or model describes the properties, characteristics, and qualities of the implementation of evidence into practice.

- *Explanatory*:   The framework or model specifies causal relationships and mechanisms of implementing evidence into practice and in relation to other phenomena.
- *Predictive*:   The framework or model predicts relationships between the dimensions or characteristics of the implementation of evidence into practice through, for example, hypotheses or propositions.

As Table 11.1 shows, the frameworks and models demonstrate a potential for one (all could be used for description), or in some case more than one purpose. These uses are summarized in more detail in the following text.

Stetler model: Identifies the properties and characteristics of the implementation of evidence into practice from a critical thinking perspective in a detailed way, in this sense it provides a descriptive model. Additionally, as this model is a planned action theory, it also has the potential for explanation; that is, it identifies the components and mechanisms that need to be linked together for implementation. As such, while not predictive, the model does prescribe the phases and processes that should occur for the application of evidence into practice.

Ottawa Model of Research Use (OMRU): Could be used as both a descriptive and/or explanatory model. As a planned action theory, it clearly details the steps, and actions within the phases that are required to implement evidence into practice, and thus provides an explanation of the processes involved. As the authors state, the prescriptiveness of the model is in the requirement to assess, monitor, and evaluate.

Promoting Action on Research Implementation in Health Services (PARIHS) framework: Has the potential to be used for description, explanation, and prediction. It describes the characteristics and properties of the successful implementation of evidence into practice. Explanation is achieved through the linkage of, and relationships between framework elements and subelements. The potential for prediction is in the identification of a number of hypotheses that could be tested about the relationships between the elements and subelements.

Iowa model of evidence-based practice: Could also be used for description and explanation. Like the Stetler and OMRU models, this is a planned action theory, which provides guidance about the steps and processes that need to take place to bring about change.

Dissemination and use of research evidence for policy and practice model: Could be used both as a descriptive and a predictive model. It describes the factors that are important in facilitating EBP. Additionally, the model has the potential to generate a number of overarching hypotheses about certain components in the model and their relationship to knowledge translation broadly – as opposed to hypotheses about the relationships between the model's components and research use.

Advancing Research and Clinical practice through close Collaboration (ARCC) model: Has the potential to be used for description and prediction. Specifically, it describes the factors that are important for the process of implementing evidence into practice. Additionally, the model facilitates the development of broad hypotheses between various elements or components of the framework.

Joanna Briggs Institute (JBI) model of evidence-based health care: Is a descriptive framework, which describes the key elements and processes involved in synthesizing and embedding evidence into practice.

Knowledge To Action (KTA) framework: Could be used as a descriptive and/or explanatory framework. The framework, based on planned action theory, describes the stages involved in the implementation of evidence into practice. Additionally, it provides an explanatory framework in that it could help its users understand the causal relationships between its different components.

In summary, clearly the models and frameworks in this book could be used for a variety of purposes. Therefore, choosing among them will be dependent on what the user wants to achieve. For example, if it is important to understand the factors that might have influenced whether implementation has been successful or not, or in planning for implementation, the factors that need attention, choosing descriptive and explanatory frameworks and/or models would be appropriate. If one is planning an implementation evaluation, such as a trial, it would be relevant to draw on frameworks and/or models that facilitate hypothesis testing. In cases where the process of implementation needs more explicit guiding, choosing one of the explanatory models that links the components of the process together would be appropriate. Of course, the decisions about application also need to be informed by the other factors and characteristics highlighted throughout this chapter.

Development

We were interested in finding out more about the development of the models and frameworks. More specifically, we applied the following questions to this analysis:

- Was the framework developed inductively or deductively?
- Was the framework/model developed from empirical and/or collective insights?
- Is there evidence to support or refute the framework/model?

With the exception of the dissemination and use of research evidence for policy and practice model, and the KTA framework, most of the models and frameworks appear to have been originally developed inductively. In some cases, over time following original conception/ conceptualization, research and development work has led to changes and refinements to some of them (e.g., Stetler model, PARIHS, Iowa, ARCC, dissemination and use of research evidence for policy and practice model). While often difficult to keep track of versions of a framework or model's developments, arguably the process of research, reflection, refinement, and continuous development could ultimately lead to a more precise and therefore more useful product.

Those models and frameworks that were developed inductively drew on a variety of sources of information in their development, but commonly, experience. For example, the developers of the Ottawa Model of Research Use drew on research, theory, and expert opinion to develop what they describe as a practical model to promote research use. Stetler describes an inductive process to the development of her original model, drawing on experience in the field. Similarly, PARIHS was originally developed from the collective wisdom and experience of the developers in quality improvement, practice development, and research. The JBI model of evidence-based health care and ARCC were also conceived from the experience of the developers within their respective organizations.

In contrast, the KTA framework was partly developed from an evidence review of planned action theories. In this process, 31 planned action theories were subject to theory analysis. Once commonalities had been identified across these theories a seven-step process was developed, which represents the action part of the framework. The content part of the framework (knowledge creation, synthesis, tools/products) was developed through consultation, reflection, and debate. The two aspects of process and content were then combined by the developers. Dobbins *et al.* also developed the initial version of the dissemination and use of research evidence for policy and practice model from a synthesis of a number of bodies of evidence including literature on organizational behavior, culture, decision making, EBP, research utilization, and dissemination.

The maturity and arguably robustness of a framework and model is in the evidence that supports or refutes it. Perhaps unsurprisingly given the different ages and stages of development of the models and frameworks included here, the developers report varying amounts of evidence to support them. Table 11.3 summarizes the evidence (excluding reference to citations) provided by the developers that

Table 11.3 Summary of framework and model use

Framework/model	Types of use	Types of evidence
Stetler model	• Formative/summative evaluations • To support EBP intervention work • Model testing • Clinical projects • Informing EBP program development within health care institutions • Informing development of curricula	• Case reports (e.g., of advanced practice nurses) • Audit • Qualitative research • Academic theses • Conference presentations
OMRU	• To guide research studies • To inform analysis • Quality improvement research and initiatives • To guide implementation projects and address clinical problems	• Qualitative research • Quantitative research • Mixed methods research • Conference presentations
PARIHS	• As a conceptual framework for research and evaluation projects (e.g., overall design, intervention development)	• Qualitative research (e.g., action research, ethnography, case study) • Quantitative research (including statistical modeling)

Table 11.3 (*Continued*)

Framework/model	Types of use	Types of evidence
	• As a basis for tool development • For modeling research utilization • As a tool to diagnose and evaluate readiness • Practice development • Student projects	• Mixed methods research • Conference presentations
Iowa	• To guide improvement projects and initiatives (e.g., pain management) • As the basis for curriculum development • As a guiding framework for grant applications • For evidence-based practice research/implementation science	• Qualitative research • Quantitative research (including large trials) • Mixed method research • Quality improvement data
Dissemination and use of research evidence for policy and practice model	• To inform the development of others' models • To inform knowledge translation and exchange strategies/interventions • To theoretically inform research studies	• Qualitative research • Quantitative research (e.g., randomized controlled trial)
ARCC	• Scale development • Intervention testing (mentor vs. no mentor) • To guide workshop development	• Qualitative and quantitative instrument development research • Pilot randomized trial
JBI model of evidence-based health care	• As an approach to guide the JBI collaboration • To inform a clinical fellow program	• Curriculum documentation
KTA	• To inform policy (Canadian Institutes for Health Research) • As a conceptual framework for research projects • As a guide for knowledge management strategy	• Policy documentation and messaging • Research proposals

PARIHS, Promoting Action on Research Implementation in Health Services; ARCC, Advancing Research and Clinical practice through close Collaboration; JBI, Joanna Briggs Institute; KTA, Knowledge To Action; OMRU, Ottowa Model for Research Use.

supports their framework/model's use. As we have used the developer's accounts to construct this summary, the reader is reminded that this may not reflect the true extent of each models/frameworks' use.

This summary demonstrates the breadth of ways these various models and frameworks have been used and therefore how they could be used in future implementation activity. Of course there will be other ways in which these frameworks and models could be used that have not been captured here. A later section in this chapter, for example, considers whether there is the potential to use models and frameworks such as these in classroom or hypothetical situations.

Theoretical underpinnings

As described in Chapter 2, frameworks and models coexist with theory. Therefore, whether the frameworks and models have explicit or implicit theoretical underpinnings, and what these are, was of interest. Our analysis shows that in most cases the theoretical underpinnings of the frameworks and models have been explicitly stated and include those listed in Table 11.4.

Two authors also make the point with their chapters (see Chapters 5 and 10) that their frameworks could also be populated by other

Table 11.4 Theoretical underpinnings of models and frameworks

Model/framework	Theoretical underpinnings
Stetler model	Planned action theory
OMRU	Rogers' Diffusion of Innovations Planned action theory
PARIHS	Diffusion of Innovations, organizational theory, and humanism
Iowa	Quality and performance improvement, organizational and systems literature
Dissemination and use of research evidence for policy and practice model	Rogers' Diffusion of Innovation
ARCC	Control Theory and Cognitive–Behavioral Theory
KTA	Planned action theories

PARIHS, Promoting Action on Research Implementation in Health Services; ARCC, Advancing Research and Clinical practice through close Collaboration; KTA, Knowledge To Action; OMRU, Ottowa Model for Research Use.

mid-range theories; this includes the PARIHS framework and the KTA framework. In both cases it is suggested that, depending on the particular objectives of an implementation effort, multiple mid-range theories (see Chapter 2 for more detail about mid-range theories) at multiple points and/or levels could be incorporated into either framework's application. This provides an example of one distinction between the utility of a framework versus a model; a framework, by virtue of the fact that it is an organized set of concepts, rather than a more prescribed and precise representation, should be able to be applied to more situations and in more flexible ways.

It is useful to know how models and frameworks are theoretically underpinned, not only from the point of view of providing evidence of its theoretical coherence, but also to facilitate decisions about appropriate application. For example, if embarking on a project that requires attention to the process of implementing a specific piece of evidence or knowledge product, selecting a model underpinned by planned action theory has the potential to provide a "road map" of the different phases or steps one would need to consider. Equally, if an objective is to better understand the factors that might influence evidence/knowledge uptake or use, then a model or framework underpinned by the theory of diffusion of innovations would be an appropriate selection. Of course, as mentioned previously there would be no reason why particular frameworks and models could not be combined, if one counteracts the deficiencies (for project purposes) of the other.

Conceptual clarity

Some of the questions that relate to a framework and/or models' conceptual coherence, robustness, and therefore usefulness, concern their conceptual clarity (see Chapter 2 for a more detailed description of these issues). Specifically, the following questions could be used to test robustness and usefulness:

- Does the framework or model have a well described and coherent language for enabling the identification of key elements?
- Does the framework or model enable the identification of similarities and differences between theories as well as their strengths and weaknesses?
- Does the framework or model have the potential to stimulate new theoretical developments?

Overall, as the previous chapters in which developers describe their models and frameworks show, the elements, concepts, and components of these have been well described. It should be clear from these descriptions (and their linked resources and references) what the constitution of each model and framework is, which should in turn facilitate their potential use.

Arguably the potential to stimulate new theoretical insights will vary, not only in relation to why each framework or model is applied (e.g., theoretical insights might not be an objective of interest in a quality improvement project), but also by how it is applied. If we take the application of the KTA framework as an example; if it is used as an overarching framework to broadly guide implementation activity and/or research, its use is unlikely to facilitate the generation of new theoretical insights, unless these emerge through inductive inquiry. However, if it is used more *specifically* to, for example, develop implementation interventions, or for the assessment of facilitators and barriers it could have more potential to generate insights. So, for example, in taking one of the stages of the framework "select, tailor, implement interventions" (see Chapter 10 for more details about the framework), applying relevant mid-range theory to this stage, such as social support theory could lead to the development of an opinion leader intervention. The implementation of the opinion leader intervention and its impact on knowledge use ("monitor knowledge use") could have the potential to shed new light on opinion leadership and therefore the theory of social support in knowledge translation. Taking the PARIHS framework as a further example; as stated in Chapter 5 one of the outstanding questions with respect to this framework is how the elements (evidence, context, and facilitation) and their subelements interrelate and interact with each other within implementation processes and to what effect. This is a theoretical question because the answer would enhance the framework's specificity. Therefore applying the question "How do evidence, context, and facilitation relate to each other" within an implementation project could stimulate new insights about the PARIHS framework. These are just two examples, all the developers of the frameworks and models in Chapters 3–10 outlined research and theoretical questions that still require consideration. Paying attention to these provides the potential to stimulate new theoretical developments about the implementation of evidence into practice.

Levels

An important question when designing an implementation strategy is to determine what level the strategy is directed toward. For example, if the evidence is related to a specific change in individual clinician behavior that effects their own patient care, then choosing a model that is targeted toward the individual may be more suitable. However, if the practice change involves multiple clinicians working together to implement a guideline in a specialist ward then the chosen model should be appropriate for a team or a unit, depending on the guideline. It may be that it is an interdisciplinary guideline in which case the model/framework chosen should be applicable across disciplines. Similarly, if the implementation strategy is focused on an organizational change or directed toward the release and implementation of a new policy on a national basis, then again model selection is important.

Table 11.2 demonstrates our analysis of the levels the models/frameworks have been developed for, and used within. For example, Stetler's model was initially developed for improving the use of evidence in practice by individuals. Later revisions of the model have successfully incorporated group level involvement where more complex changes are necessary across the whole unit not just by individuals. As described in Chapter 1, the focus on individuals was not uncommon in early research with little attention given to the role and impact of the team on the success of implementation, unit leadership or even hospital policies. More commonly, we now see models/frameworks that offer flexibility for targeting different levels depending on the need and the evidence to be implemented.

Nevertheless, few of the models/frameworks are designed to encompass change at the policy level. The use of the dissemination and use of research evidence for policy and practice model in policy implementation studies is likely to be related to its origins from the management field and Diffusion of Innovations Theory. The KTA Framework has been created for use by both researchers creating the knowledge and end users implementing the knowledge. The design incorporates multiple levels that can occur independently or simultaneously. Similarly, PARIHS offers a broad framework suitable for use at team level upwards.

Although most models can be used at the individual level, three of them appear not to be applicable, PARIHS, dissemination and use of research evidence for policy and practice model, and JBI model of evidence-based health care. In the case of PARIHS, it has not included any elements concerning the individual's knowledge and skills in implementing evidence into practice. This is possibly related to the level of detail some frameworks offer as a way of organizing thinking, rather than the precise detail offered by others that are planned action theories. As can be seen in Table 11.2, nearly all models/frameworks work at several levels (see Table 11.2 for specific areas of relevance for each model/framework).

Situation

In response to global workforce shortages in all health professions, growing numbers of health professional students are being educated. As a consequence of growth in the sector, increased clinical placements are necessary for students to gain clinical experience and exposure to real-world problems and contexts. However, it is not always possible for clinical settings to provide enough access for students for the number of placements needed. This international problem has forced educators and academics to think more broadly about alternate delivery modes traditionally delivered in the clinical setting. This includes educating students in the processes necessary for engaging in EBP. Students require either clinical practice experience or an opportunity to learn through simulation or hypothetical cases.

While an actual dynamic clinical experience offers an opportunity to learn in changing contexts, adjusting barriers and enablers, and shifting social interactions; all of which are known to impact on the implementation process. Studies taking place in clinical practice, although unpredictable, offers significant opportunity for discovery of new knowledge and greater understanding. However, the ability to use models and frameworks in hypothetical situations offers greater control over experimentation, that is specific contextual elements can be scheduled or programd to challenge learners on using evidence in a controlled situation. Similar to problem-based learning situations, hypothetical cases could be used in a controlled situation where role modeling and problem solving were demonstrated.

For this reason, we wanted to review the types of situations that the models and frameworks could be used in to teach clinicians' and students' approaches to implementing evidence into practice.

There was no doubt that all these models had been used in a variety of clinical settings. What is less clear is whether these models and frameworks could be used with hypothetical cases. There was some evidence of models being used in curriculums or student projects that indicated a potential for simulated use (e.g., Iowa, Stetler, ARCC). However, it was unclear from the text what specific circumstances the models/frameworks had been used in these areas. The developers of the Stetler model, Iowa model, and the dissemination and use of research evidence for policy and practice model specifically noted undergraduate and graduate use, and the design of training and internship curricula.

Users

Health care environments are information-rich organizations, where health professionals by necessity are required to work together; communicating with others from different disciplines to share information about patients, to plan, organize, deliver, and evaluate individual patient care. Even in areas such as primary care where clinicians may work independently, they often need to communicate with external providers for services not available within their organization. To increase applicability for different user groups, the majority of models are designed to be used by interdisciplinary groups. In addition, some of them are sufficiently amenable and generic in terminology, that they could also be used outside the health care sector.

As previously mentioned, most of the models were developed inductively, from within acute health care settings where the largest group of professionals employed are nurses. For this reason, it is not surprising that the models and frameworks highlighted in this text have been developed by nurses or by teams including nurses for nursing practice improvement. (For a summary of other interdisciplinary models and frameworks not featured in this book, see Appendix.)

Stetler's model evolved from the author's nursing experience as a way of guiding nurses in the process of research utilization. Similarly, the ARCC model and JBI model of evidence-based health care also evolved from nursing experience in implementing EBP changes for nursing care. Both the Stetler model and ARCC specifically recognized the knowledge and skills of advanced practice nurses as being requisite for facilitating EBP. Both of these models targeted advanced practice nurses in mentoring roles to change the culture of units and organizations. The Iowa model is a team approach that requires critical synthesis of research literature as part of the model. So although it is not limited to advanced practice nurses, the process would usually involve nurses with higher education skills to be working on the team to facilitate the synthesis of research for practice.

In contrast, the dissemination and use of research evidence for policy and practice model and KTA framework were deductively developed from syntheses of literature both within and outside health care literature. This external influence has lead to more generic terminology, which possibly enhances their applicability across users groups. Table 11.5 below summarizes the potential users for each model and framework.

Function

In reviewing the chapters describing the different models, it was clear that the functions varied between the models and frameworks, and that these offered some distinguishing features that would assist user choice depending on their needs. Four specific functions were identified:

- Assessment of facilitators and barriers.
- Intervention development.
- Outcome measurement and variable selection.
- Evaluation of processes.

Table 11.5 User application of models and frameworks

Model/framework	Potential users
Stetler model	Nurses
OMRU	All clinicians
PARIHS	All clinicians
Iowa model of evidence-based practice	All clinicians
Dissemination and use of research evidence for policy and practice model	All clinicians and policy makers
ARCC	Nurses
JBI model of evidence-based health care	Nurses and allied health
KTA	All clinicians and policy makers

PARIHS, Promoting Action on Research Implementation in Health Services; ARCC, Advancing Research and Clinical practice through close Collaboration; JBI, Joanna Briggs Institute; KTA, Knowledge To Action; OMRU, Ottowa Model for Research Use.

Table 11.2 illustrates the different functions pertaining to each model/framework.

As implementation researchers and clinicians have begun to understand the importance of context in influencing the likely success of implementation, *assessment of barriers and facilitators* as a diagnostic tool prior to implementation has become recognized as critical to the success of the intervention or strategy. Some frameworks, such as PARIHS, use explicit terminology and comprise the dimensions of culture, leadership, and evaluation. A conducive context for EBP is stated to be one in which roles are clear, staff are valued, where there is decentralized decision making, transformational leadership and the use of multiple indicators on performance (Rycroft-Malone, 2008).

All models and frameworks with the exception of the Iowa model included some form of contextual analysis. Stetler specifically refers to the three R's; risk, resources, and readiness. ARCC, JBI, OMRU, and KTA all refer to assessment of barriers and facilitators. Dissemination and use of research evidence for policy and practice model under the element persuasion refers to the individual and organizational characteristics preceding the decision-making process.

Sales *et al.* (2006) have argued that understanding the barriers and facilitators enables a more targeted selection of interventions to maximize the success; implying the contextual analysis is one of the preliminary steps in the implementation process. A diagnostic assessment offers the opportunity to counter barriers and to build on the enablers. Ploeg *et al.* (2007) have identified barriers and facilitators at each level from the individual level through to the organizational level determinants.

The second function pertains to *intervention development*. All models and frameworks either stated explicit functions in developing the intervention (Iowa, KTA, Stetler, and OMRU) or had developed a variety of tools associated with various elements such as a facilitation toolkit (PARIHS) or clinical audit (JBI). Two models/frameworks had the intervention development embedded (ARCC and dissemination and use of research evidence for policy and practice model). ARCC focuses on the use of EBP mentors as the intervention in facilitating the evidence through the organization, the specific way the intervention was managed depended on the organizational assessment.

Measurement of outcomes is a critical component of health care. Evaluating the evidence forms a key function to substantiate the continuation, change, or cessation of clinical practices. Selection of the appropriate variables is the starting point for measuring the success of the intervention. Most models identified variable selection for outcome measurement as a required step in the process; some were more prescriptive than others; such as the Iowa model that identifies measurement of process and outcomes. Others such as KTA were more implicit, possibly because the detail of measurement is more likely to be found in the original research rather than the synthesis framework. See Table 11.2 for specific models and frameworks with this function.

The final function we identified was the *evaluation of processes*. All models and frameworks were unequivocal in the identification of process evaluation as a step in implementation. For example, the KTA phase of "evaluate outcomes" contains the construct of process evaluation. JBI evaluates the process outcomes and the impact on the system. Iowa refers to "Monitor and analyze structure, process and outcome data." Similarly, OMRU monitors intervention use and measures outcomes. In the dissemination and use of research evidence for policy and practice model, there is a significant construct dedicated to the confirmation phase. It has a role in determining the success of the innovation adoption outlining examples of the process and outcome measures available to the consumer. Likewise for Stetler's model, a whole phase is dedicated to evaluation of process and outcome measures. PARIHS has the subelement evaluation as part of the context. In contrast, the ARCC model is more implicit in that it refers to the use of EBP mentors to achieve an EBP organizational culture that will lead to quality patient outcomes, staff related outcomes, and decreased cost rather than it being part of the implementation process to measure process and outcomes.

Testable

For the final dimension, we were curious about the models and frameworks' ability to generate testable hypotheses and/or propositions. We also wanted to establish if the model/framework was supported by empirical data. From the authors' descriptions, we acknowledge that most of the models and frameworks were testable and had supporting empirical evidence (see Table 11.2 for our findings about this function). Most authors offered hypotheses that clearly identified propositions that successful implementation was moderated by the various elements within the model to a greater or lesser extent.

As examples of hypotheses testing, Dobbins *et al.* (2009) had tested the dissemination and use of research evidence for policy and practice model on hypotheses concerning the impact of organizational characteristics on knowledge translation. The PARIHS team have also begun testing the construct facilitation while other researchers (Cummings *et al.*, 2007) have used empirical methods to measure the association between organizational characteristics (context as defined and described in the PARIHS model) and research utilization.

As the most established model, Stetler described significant empirical work that she has completed in validating the model, as well as offering further opportunities for testing assumptions (see Table 3.2). Like the Iowa model, it was developed as a practice model rather than a research model. Stetler outlines numerous published uses of the model and distinguishes between use and evaluation of the model. The prescriptive nature of the model provides practitioners with greater stepwise detail and thus is more likely to be acceptable by clinicians for implementation in clinical settings. Several of the authors have described developments as evolving from practice, as opposed to those developed from knowledge synthesis. This may be an interesting distinction between the models and frameworks when determining those most useful for researchers, and those most practical for clinicians.

Nevertheless, hypotheses and propositions have been generated in most models and frameworks regardless of their origins. The type and quantity of empirical research conducted on each model/framework appears partly related to maturity (i.e., their age) but is also related to the logic and intuitive feel of some. Sometimes the flexibility offered by a conceptual framework may mean it is more amenable to research testing. Whereas a more prescriptive model may mean that elements appear so complex so as to make the research context too intricate to study in anything but an observational approach.

The author's descriptions of the empirical work being conducted on the various models and frameworks are reported in earlier chapters. In terms of methodological approaches, Table 11.3 demonstrates the various ways and designs that have been reported for each model/framework. The table highlights the breadth of methods used and available to study the implementation process. Following the general rule that the question will determine the method, the investigation of implementation interventions and strategies to increase our understanding may require an eclectic response and openness to new methods. As discussed in Chapter 2, different theories will propagate different levels of understanding.

Conclusion

This chapter has presented our analysis of the models and frameworks described in Chapters 3–10 by their developers. To assist us in this task, we developed a framework that included key dimensions related to robustness and application. We made a judgment about each framework and model based on these criteria, which also informed the narrative synthesis described in the preceding sections. As we stated earlier, our motivation for applying these criteria was not to make a value judgment about the worth of each model or framework, rather, our aim was to summarize some of their qualities so that readers could use this information to make their own informed choices.

As our analysis and synthesis shows many of the individual models and frameworks could be used in different situations, for different purposes, and with different users. Therefore, matching the particular requirements of an evidence into practice project, to the various qualities of the frameworks and models should be relatively straightforward. It is also helpful to note not only how the developers perceive their frameworks and models *could* be used, but also how others *have* used them, which includes a breadth of examples from quality improvement to modeling research use.

We also hope that the criteria that we have developed will be useful to the assessment of other models and frameworks, not included in this book. Using them should help determine the best fit, which of course should not preclude the use of more than one framework or model to guide or underpin a single initiative.

References

Cummings, G.G., Estabrooks, C.A., Midodzi, W.K., Wallin, L., Hayduk, L. (2007). Influence of organizational characteristics and context on research utilization. *Nursing Research*, 56: S25–S39.

Dobbins, M., Hanna, S., Ciliska, D., Thomas, H., Manske, S., Cameron, R., *et al.* (2009). A randomized controlled trial evaluating the impact of knowledge transfer and exchange strategies. *Implementation Science*, 4:61.

Ploeg, J., Davies, B., Edwards, N., Gifford, W., and Elliot Miller, P. (2007). Factors influencing best-practice guideline implementation: Lessons learned from administrators, nursing staff, and project leaders. *Worldviews on Evidence-Based Nursing*, 4:210–219.

Rycroft-Malone, J. (2008). Evidence-informed practice: From individual to context. *Journal of Nursing Management*, 16(4):404–408 (Special Issue).

Sales, A., Smith, J., Curran, G., and Kochevar, L. (2006). Models, strategies, and tools. Theory in implementing evidence-based findings into health care practice. *Journal of General Internal Medicine*, 21:S21–S24.

Chapter 12

Summary and concluding comments

Jo Rycroft-Malone and Tracey Bucknall

This final chapter picks up the threads that we began at the start of this book; particularly in relation to the complexities of implementing evidence in practice. We then consider some broader issues about the use of models and frameworks in implementation work, before presenting specific examples of applications as illustrations. Finally we outline some ongoing challenges and make links to the other books in this evidence-based practice implementation series.

A note about implementation

Our aim with this book is to provide a resource to facilitate the process(es) involved in the implementation of evidence in practice by using theory, models, and frameworks. We therefore began by setting out a context that highlighted the complexities of implementing evidence in practice, where evidence is defined in a broad or pluralistic sense. Policy mechanisms, such as guideline development organizations, are predicated on an assumption that evidence use is something that automatically happens once a guideline has been published and disseminated. However, it has now been recognized that "pushing out" or disseminating research information has only limited success (Nutley *et al.*, 2003). Some early models that describe implementation of evidence into practice did promote this linear process where the emphasis was on informing and monitoring, with a view to changing practice. However, while slow, there has been a shift to recognize that in fact the process of implementing evidence in practice is more complex, involving social, organizational, as well as individual factors (e.g., Dopson and Fitzgerald 2005; Dopson *et al.*, 2003; Nutely *et al.*, 2007). Chapter 1 described some of the components and influences of evidence-based practice in more detail.

A systematic review of the diffusion of innovations literature (Greenhalgh *et al.*, 2004) adds further emphasis to this argument by introducing the analogy of a "contact sport." While the diffusion of innovations is not necessarily synonymous with the implementation of evidence into practice, the findings from the review are relevant to increasing our understanding of the many factors that might be important in whether evidence is used or not. The analogy of a "contact sport" was further developed by Rycroft-Malone (2005) in which it is suggested that implementing evidence in practice necessitates the challenge, negotiation, and overcoming of various boundaries, objects, and players:

> In a contact sport such as ice hockey or rugby, the interaction between a number of different elements determines the nature of the game, the spirit in which it is played, and the ultimate outcome – win or lose. The same could be said of getting evidence into practice: It is the interaction of various ingredients that determines the success of the outcome
>
> —Rycroft-Malone, 2005: 1.

Despite the acknowledgment that using evidence is complex and multifaced, for some time there has been a focus on developing the skills and knowledge of *individual* practitioner's to appraise research and make rationale decisions; with questionable success – for the most part research evidence is not routinely used in practice. We acknowledge that ultimately individuals are the decision makers; however within the health care setting, individuals can not be isolated from the influence of all the other bureaucratic, political, organizational, and social factors that affect change and adoption of new practices. The implementation of research-based practice depends on an ability to achieve significant and planned change involving individuals, teams, and organizations. People are not passive recipients of evidence; rather they are stakeholders in problem-solving processes, which are social and interactional. This complexity has led some to suggest that practice can only ever be evidence-informed, rather than evidence-based (Davies *et al.*, 2000).

Nutely *et al.* (2007) provide an excellent synthesis of the factors that shape evidence use across the public services more broadly. Their analysis results in a number of guiding principles for the use of research in practice, which is summarized in Table 12.1 (see Nutely *et al.*, 2007: 312 for their interpretation).

Table 12.1 Guiding principles for the use of evidence in practice

Guiding principles	Explanation
Research needs to be translated	Research shows that evidence is socially and historically constructed. That is, a piece of research evidence is likely to mean different things to different groups, and individuals. Additionally, research tends to get transformed in the process of use – research evidence is rarely used as presented, in for example, guidelines. Therefore undertaking adaptation processes are likely to make research findings more usable, including tailoring, packaging, and consensus development.
Ownership is critical	Ownership in relation to the research itself or the implementation process is likely to affect uptake. Exceptions to this would be system based, top–down approaches that "force" research use through an organization's systems and processes.
Enthusiasts are key	People who are enthusiastic about the issue/topic/practice change can act as champions and sell new ideas.
Conduct an analysis of context	An analysis of the context of implementation prior to designing implementation processes/strategies can facilitate more particularized approaches through the targeting of barriers and facilitators.
Ensure credibility	Research use is enhanced by credible evidence, credible champions/opinion leaders, and a commitment to process.
Provide leadership	Strong and facilitative leaders at project and organizational levels can lend strategic support and potential integration, space, resources, and authority to the process.
Provide adequate support/resources	Implementation needs adequate resources and support including financial, human (e.g., dedicated project leaders), and appropriate equipment.
Develop opportunities for integration	Activities, changes, and new practices need to be integrated into an organization's systems and processes to enhance the potential of their sustainability. Initiatives that fit with strategic priorities are more likely to be given/allocated adequate resources and support.

From Nutely *et al.* (2007).

Previous chapters in this book have described, to various extents, how factors such as those outlined in Table 12.1 might influence implementation and how to overcome them through the application of particular models and frameworks, and/or their constituent parts.

A note about impact

At this point it is also worth highlighting that (research) evidence can impact in different ways. Therefore the choice of model or framework to facilitate an implementation process may be influenced by what needs to be achieved. Research can impact through *instrumental use*: the direct impact of research/knowledge on practice and policy; *conceptual use*: how knowledge may impact on thinking, understanding, and attitudes; and *symbolic use*: how knowledge may be used as a political tool to legitimatize opposition or practice (after Weiss, 1979, see Fig. 12.1). So, research evidence (e.g., guideline recommendations) can have a more or less direct impact on practice and/or policy. The gap between behavior or practice; and how a change in practice or behavior then translates into a change in (patient) outcomes is notoriously challenging to achieve, evaluate, and measure. That is, changes in behavior or practice may not necessarily result in a change to patient outcomes (instrumental use). See Fig. 12.2 for an example of how different types of impact can be embedded within the application of a framework.

The evidence-based practice movement has focused attention on influencing instrumental impact, that is, making a difference to patient outcomes. However, it is worth remembering that to have an instrumental impact, it is likely that (in many cases) other types of impact need to accumulate to eventually make an impact on summative outcomes.

Therefore in choosing a model or framework, decision making may be guided by the sort of impact you are interested in making.

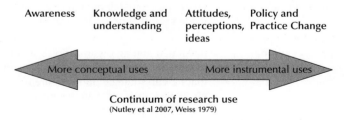

Figure 12.1 Types of impact (after Nutley *et al.*, 2007; Weiss 1979)

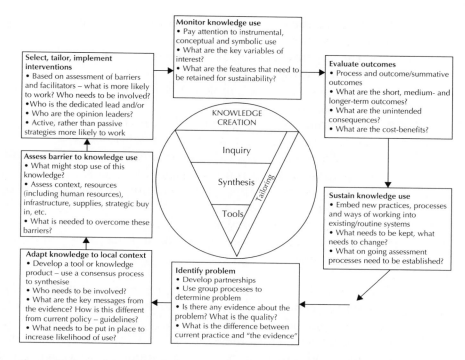

Figure 12.2 Applying Knowledge To Action (KTA) to implementation: An example

For example, if raising an individual practitioner's awareness of an issue and/or increasing their knowledge and understanding about an issue is important, it would seem sensible to consider applying a model or framework that pays attention to these individual level factors (e.g., Stetler, Iowa, ARCC, OMRU).

Applying models and frameworks to guide implementation

The models and frameworks in this book provide some guiding principles, rather than recipes for success for facilitating the implementation of evidence into practice. As Chapter 2 outlined there are a number of ways that models and frameworks can be used in implementation activity (both practice and research), which are summarized in the following list.

- At a broad level, to provide a frame of reference:
  - for organizing thinking;
  - as a guide for what to focus on;
  - for interpretation and better understanding.

- To guide the choice and development of interventions/implementation strategies:
  - for targeting participants/groups;
  - for assessing barriers and facilitators;
  - for planning the implementation process(es) and targeting change efforts.
- To facilitate an appropriate choice of tools and measurement devices, and focus on relevant variables of interest.
- To direct the user toward appropriate implementation and evaluation approaches/methodologies and methods.
- To guide the use of appropriate mid-range theories (if appropriate).
- To facilitate the development of new knowledge, insights, and theory (both inductively and deductively).
- To increase the chances of a successful outcome – impact, that is, using evidence in practice.

They have the potential to be helpful in these ways because they contain the concepts, components and in some cases, processes that need to be attended to if the chances of successful implementation are to be increased. How these model and framework concepts, components, and processes should be applied and enacted has been described by their developers in Chapters 3–10.

Chapter 2 also described what makes a conceptual framework or model coherent, robust and therefore potentially more useful. Our view is that there is little point using a framework or model for implementation if, fundamentally, it is not robust. We translated these criteria into a number of dimensions that we used to make an assessment of the descriptions of the various models and frameworks described in this book. As we stated in Chapter 11 it was not our intention to make a value judgment about how the frameworks and models measured up to these criteria; readers can make an assessment from the information in Table 11.1 and accompanying narrative. As these criteria were developed from the literature about theory and models they are transferable and could therefore be used to make an assessment about the robustness of other models and frameworks not included here (see Table 2.4).

Similarly we developed criteria to make an assessment about the application of the frameworks and models. Specifically this included at what level they could be applied, in what situations, by whom, how, and whether they are testable (see Table 2.4). Again, these criteria could be used to help make an appropriate choice about the application of other frameworks and/or models. Equally, readers may disagree with some of the judgments we have made and could use these criteria to reinterpret our summary and narrative (see Table 2.5).

Specific examples of application

A number of the model and framework developers outline application aspects within their chapters. For example, Cheryl Stetler provides an illustration of how her model could be used to the various planned action theory phases (Fig. 3.1). At each stage she includes cues to help the users make decisions about whether to proceed or consider other options. Melnyk and Fineout-Overholt also identify a number of tools and measures that could be used as part of the ARCC model's application. Additionally the examples that contributors have included of others' use of their frameworks and models will provide useful follow-up information.

The various models and frameworks could also be tailored for use. It is likely that in most cases frameworks and models would need to be particularized for the specifics of a project/initiative. We have provided two examples by way of illustration. Box 12.1 illustrates how the core concepts and elements of the PARIHS framework can be converted into a set of questions that could be used as a checklist when embarking on an implementation project.

Similarly, Fig. 12.2 provides an example of an application of the Knowledge To Action (KTA) framework based on *our* interpretation of the framework and knowledge of implementation.

While not within the explicit remit of this book, some contributing authors also highlighted that their models and frameworks had been used within education settings or as part of the development of curricula for workshops and other training events. Our synthesis framework included an assessment of each model and framework's potential to be used both hypothetically (e.g., within a classroom setting or simulated environment) and in "real" situations (i.e., practice environments or settings) (refer to Chapter 11 for more information). The interest in simulation within education contexts is increasing (e.g., Melnyk, 2008). Therefore it will be interesting to see whether over time more prominence will be given within classroom settings on how to use and apply evidence-based practice frameworks and models more broadly, rather than focusing on certain components of some of them as commonly happens now (e.g., critical appraisal of evidence).

Box 12.1 Applying PARIHS to implementation: an example

Evidence

- Is there any research evidence underpinning the initiative/topic?
- Is this research judged to be well conceived, designed, and conducted?
- Are the findings from research relevant to the initiative/topic?
- What is the practitioner's experience and opinion about this topic and the research evidence?
- Does the research evidence match clinical experience?
- If it does not, why might this be so?
- Do you need to seek consensus before it might be used by practitioners in this setting?
- What is the patient's experience/preference/story concerning this initiative/topic?
- Does this differ from practitioners' perspectives?
- How could a partnership approach be developed?
- Is there any robust, local information/data about the initiative/topic?
- Would it be appropriate to develop a knowledge/evidence product that combines all these types of evidence?

Context

- Is the context of implementation receptive to change?
- What are the beliefs and values of the organization, team, and practice context?
- What sort of leadership style is present (command and control – transformational)?
- Are individual and team boundaries clear?
- Is there effective team working (inter and multidisciplinary)?
- Does evaluation of performance rely on broad and varied sources of information?
- Is this information fed back to clinical contexts?

Facilitation

- Consider the answers to the evidence and context questions: what are the barriers and what are the facilitators to this initiative?
- What tasks/activities and processes require facilitation?
- Given the people and setting, what sort of skills and attributes will the person facilitating require to be effective in the role?
- Would it be appropriate to draw on the skills and knowledge of an external facilitator to work with internal facilitators?
- What role might the facilitator have in evaluating the outcomes of the project?

Before moving on, it is probably worth reiterating the distinction between using frameworks and models to guide implementation science/research, and using them to inform or guide the implementation of research evidence in practice settings. Our main focus in this book was on the latter goal: to facilitate the application of models and frameworks in guiding the implementation of evidence in practice. However, many of the issues covered in the book will likely be relevant to both their use in practice, and their use in research, particularly in relation to, for example, developing theory (including practice theory) from implementation activity. We therefore expect that the included contributions stimulate future research and development work, as many of the authors highlighted where there are gaps in knowledge.

Concluding remarks

Within this book we have brought together a collection of models and frameworks that might facilitate the implementation of evidence-based practice, however, there is still much to learn about implementation and about how best to apply these types of organizing devices to those activities. Some of the frameworks and models have undergone substantial use and have developed over time, others are younger and will continue to undergo testing and further refinement. Additionally and more broadly, greater attention needs to be paid to the development (and testing) of theory-based interventions/strategies, that is, interventions and strategies that have an increased chance of making an impact by virtue of the fact they are theoretically and evidentially sound. The application of theoretically robust and conceptually coherent models and frameworks should facilitate these endeavors. There is a good rationale for using these types of heuristics; they can help to make sense of implementation by guiding the process, and by focusing attention on the important things. Just like evidence needs to be tailored before being used, frameworks and models are also likely to require some particularization; they should facilitate, not constrain implementation efforts.

The selection and application of a framework or model should come early in the process; it should be the foundation upon which implementation projects and initiatives are built. There are also other important considerations, which are considered by other books in this implementation series.

The complexities of implementation were outlined in the preceding text and described in more detail in Chapter 1. This included the idea that implementation is likely to be partly dependant on the nature of context and/or contextual factors. There has been a growing awareness of the importance of context and how it might impact on or mediate the implementation and use of evidence in practice, for this reason, the context of implementation is the subject of one of the other books in the series (Kent and McCormack, 2010). Within their book, Kent and McCormack, with contributions from other international authors consider how context can exert a positive or negative influence on practice environments and impact on evidence-based practice. More specifically they explore this issue by taking a look at a number of different health care contexts, for example, primary care, acute care, surgery, mental health, midwifery and aged care. From these perspectives the editors summarize the contextual issues that need to be considered when assessing the implementation of evidence-based practice and practice change.

Equally, the other book in the implementation series focuses our attention on another important issue: measuring the impact of the implementation of evidence-based practice (Bick and Graham, 2010). As Bick and Graham point out, and as we outlined earlier in this chapter, traditionally, impact has been measured by focusing on whether or not a specific clinical outcome was achieved (instrumental impact). Broader considerations of impact (which may not occur immediately) are frequently neglected (e.g. types of conceptual or symbolic impact). Their book, which also includes contributions from international authors, addresses how to identify, evaluate, and assess a broad range of outcomes of evidence use and implementation using specific examples as illustrations.

In closing we would like to revisit the premise for the development of this book; our ability to translate knowledge into practice continues to be slow, challenging and quite often, unsuccessful. That is because the issues inherent in evidence implementation and use are complex, reflecting social and interactive processes. The models and frameworks in this book help us begin to think about the ways in which we can improve evidence use because they capture and map out some of these complexities. Their application to implementation efforts will not guarantee success, but they should go some way to improving the chances.

References

Bick, D., and Graham, I. (2010). *Evaluating the impact of implementing Evidence-Based Practice*. Oxford: Blackwell Publishing.

Davies, H.T.O., Nutley, S., and Smith, P. (2000). *What Works? Evidence-Based Policy and Practice in Public Services*. London: Policy Press.

Dopson, S. and Fitzgerald, L. (eds) (2005). *Knowledge to Action? Evidence-Based Health Care in Context*. Oxford: Oxford University Press.

Dopson, S., Locock, L., Gabbay, J., Ferlie, E., and Fitzgerald, L. (2003). Evidence-based medicine and the implementation gap. *Health,* 7(3), 311–330.

Greenhalgh, T., Robert, G., Bate, P., Kyriakidou, O., Macfarlane, F., and Peacock, R. (2004). *How to Spread Good Ideas. A Systematic Review of the Literature on Diffusion, Dissemination and Sustainability of Innovations in Health Service Delivery and Organisation*. London: National Co-ordinating Centre for NHS Service Delivery and Organisation. Available at: http://www.sdo.lshtm.ac.uk.

Kent, B., and McCormack, B. (2010). *Clinical Context for Evidence-Based Practice*. Oxford: Blackwell Publishing.

Melnyk, B. (2008). Evidence to support the use of patient simulation to enhance clinical practice skills and competence in health care professionals and students. *Worldviews on Evidence-Based Nursing,* 5(1), 49–52.

Nutley, S., Walter, I., and Davies, H.T.O. (2003). From knowing to doing. A framework for understanding the evidence-into-practice agenda. *Evaluation,* 9(2), 125–148.

Nutely, S., Walters, I., and Davies, H.T.O. (2007). *Using Evidence. How Research Can Inform Public Services*. Bristol, UK: Policy Press.

Rycroft-Malone, J. (2005). Getting evidence into practice: A contact sport. *Worldviews on Evidence-Based Nursing,* 2(1), 1–3.

Weiss, C.H. (1979). The many meanings of research utilization. *Public Administration Review,* 39(5), 426–431.

Appendix
Implementation frameworks and models

	Year	Implementation framework/model	Reference
1.	1978	Western Interstate Commission for Higher Education (WICHE)	Krueger, J. C. (1978). Utilization of nursing research: The planning process. *Journal of Nursing Administration, 8*(1), 6–9.
2.	1983	Conduct and Utilisation of Research in Nursing (CURN) Project	Horsley, J. A., and Pelz, D. C. (1983). *Using Research to Improve Nursing Practice: A Guide*. San Francisco, CA: Grune & Stratton.
3.	1973	Linkage Model	Havelock, R. G. (1986). Linkage: Key to understanding the knowledge system. In G. M. Beal, W. Dissanayake, and S. Konoshima (eds), *Knowledge Generation, Exchange and Utilization*. Boulder, CO: Westview.
4.	1987	Goode Research Utilization Model	Goode, C. J., Lovett, M. K., Hayes, J. E., and Butcher, L. A. (1987). Use of research based knowledge in clinical practice. *The Journal of Nursing Administration, 17*(12), 11–18.
			Goode, C. and Bulechek, G. M. (1992). Research utilisation: An organizational process that enhances quality of care. *Journal of Nursing Care Quality: Special Report*, 27–35.
5.	1987	The Quality Assurance Model Using Research	Watson, C. A., Bulechek, G. M., and McCloskey, J. C. (1987). QAMUR: A quality assurance model using research. *Journal of Nursing Quality Assurance, 2*(1), 21–27.

(Continued)

	Year	Implementation framework/model	Reference
6.	1993	Coordinated Implementation Model	Lomas, J. (1993). Retailing research: Increasing the role of evidence in clinical services for childbirth. *The Milbank Quarterly, 71*(3), 439–475.
7.	1994	Retrieval and Application of Research in Nursing (RARIN) Model	Bostrom, J., and Wise, L. (1994). Closing the gap between research and practice. *Journal of Nursing Administration, 24*(5), 22–27.
8.	1999	Model for Change to Evidence-Based Practice	Rosswurm, M. A., and Larrabee, J. H. (1999). A model for change to Evidence-Based Practice. *Journal of Nursing Scholarship, 31*(4), 317–322.
9.	2004	ACE Star Model of Knowledge Transformation©	Stevens, K. R. (2004). *ACE Star Model of EBP: Knowledge Transformation*. Retrieved on 18 August, 2009, from www.acestar.uthscsa.edu
10.	2004	Tyler Collaborative Research Utilization Model	Olade, R. A. (2004). Strategic collaborative model for evidence-based nursing practice. *Worldviews on Evidence-based Nursing, 1*(1), 60–68.
11.	2007	Conceptual Model for Growing Evidence-Based Practice	Vratny, A., and Shriver, D. (2007). A conceptual model for growing Evidence-Based Practice. *Nursing Administration Quarterly, 31*(2), 162–170.
12.	2007	Johns Hopkins Nursing Evidence-Based Practice Model	Newhouse, R. P., Dearholt, S. L., Poe, S. S., Pugh, L. C., and White, K. M. (2007). *Johns Hopkins Nursing Evidence-Based Practice Model and Guidelines*. Indianapolis, IN: Sigma Theta Tau International Honor Society of Nursing.
13.	2008	Evidence-Based Practice Model for Staff Nurses	Reavy, K., and Tavernier, S. (2008). Nurses reclaiming ownership of their practice: implementation of an evidence-based practice model and process. *Journal of Continuing Education in Nursing, 39*(4), 166–172.

Index